Building Competence in Mindfulness-Based Cognitive Therapy

Mindfulness-based cognitive therapy (MBCT) is an evidence-based program that combines mindfulness and cognitive therapy techniques for working with stress, anxiety, depression, and other problems. *Building Competence in Mindfulness-Based Cognitive Therapy* provides the first transcript of an entire 8-week program. This intimate portrayal of the challenges and celebrations of actual clients gives the reader an inside look at the processes that occur within these groups. The author also provides insights and practical suggestions for building personal and professional competence in delivering the MBCT protocol.

"There's nothing like watching an expert in action. In this wonderfully illustrative and openhearted book, Richard Sears shares his wisdom and experience by providing a complete transcript of an 8-week course of MBCT. Whether you're an experienced provider or a novice, you'll love seeing how Dr. Sears does this. When it resembles how you do it, you'll feel validated. When it's different, you'll appreciate the fresh ideas. The introductory chapters provide insights about numerous clinical and practical issues. Both students and seasoned experts will pore over this unique book." *Ruth Baer, PhD, author of* The Practicing Happiness Workbook *and* Mindfulness-based Treatment Approaches

"Being an MBCT therapist may ask more of us than some other modes of therapy, but also may give us more in return. In particular, the need to cultivate one's own mindfulness practice can be personally challenging and also profoundly life changing. Although what we teach must be grounded in our personal practice of mindfulness, facilitating mindful awareness in others requires other skills as well (such as conducting postpractice inquiries with awareness, empathy, and compassion). Dr. Sears has given us an essential resource to help professionals become more reflective, observant, and attuned MBCT therapists. Both novice clinicians learning to facilitate MBCT groups and seasoned clinicians wishing to deepen their skills will definitely want to read this book." *Randye J. Semple, PhD, assistant professor, University of Southern California, coauthor of* Mindfulness-Based Cognitive Therapy for Anxious Children

"This book is a timely addition to the discussion about building competence in MBCT. Dr. Sears has beautifully described the process of leading participants through the 8-week program and at the same time offers useful and practical guidance about what is involved in teaching MBCT. I will recommend this book to all the MBCT trainees I teach." *Susan Woods, MSW, LICSW, senior MBSR/MBCT professional trainer, principal curriculum consultant, Mindfulness-Based Professional Training Institute, Center for Mindfulness, UC San Diego*

"Whilst the empirical literature on MBCT has been rapidly expanding in recent years, the literature on MBCT clinical practice and pedagogy has been much slower to develop. This is not surprising. MBCT teaching and learning is a subtle and delicate process which is best discovered through direct experience. However, it is wonderful to have other entry points and windows to support discovery. This valuable book offers us the opportunity of a fly-on-the-wall perspective of the intimate work that takes place within an MBCT class and the chance to join the teacher and participants in their journey through the 8 weeks. A wonderful resource for all in the field." *Rebecca Crane, Director, Centre for Mindfulness Research and Practice, Bangor University, UK*

"Richard Sears has created a rich and timely resource for anyone working in mindfulness-based interventions. This practical and thorough guide provides coverage of an MBCT course from the beginning preparations, including marketing and setting up a group space, to an inside session-by-session look at the course. With its sound examples and advice regarding important issues and specific skills invaluable to the MBI facilitator, this book will become a favorite go-to for clinicians, students, and supervisors." *Sarah Bowen, PhD, author of* Mindfulness-Based Relapse Prevention for Addictive Behaviors: A Clinician's Guide

"Leading an MBCT group is a product of a unique, personal integration of the teacher's mindfulness meditation practice with the structured MBCT protocol. Dr. Sears provides a detailed, personal example of how this integration can unfold as well as answering many common 'nuts and bolts' questions about how to facilitate an MBCT group. As such, this book is a valuable complement to the MBCT treatment manual. It will be of use to all those interested in facilitating MBCT groups, particularly for those early on in their development." *Mark A. Lau, PhD, Vancouver CBT Centre and clinical associate professor of psychiatry, University of British Columbia*

"Fascinating. Insightful. Powerful. Practical. *Building Competence in Mindfulness-Based Cognitive Therapy* is the perfect companion book for experienced or neophyte clinicians who lead MBCT, or any structured mindfulness-based group for that matter. As someone who has led hundreds of MBCT and other mindfulness-based groups, I found myself constantly learning new angles, areas of inquiry, and nuanced approaches. I commend Dr. Sears for not only his bravery in putting forth transcripts of his group sessions but also for his mindful approach that embodies wisdom, curiosity, and kindness, crucial qualities for us to practice and express in mindfulness groups. I am confident that those who give these chapters a careful reading, with a mindset toward application, will find themselves more confident, comfortable, and socially tuned in during their own mindfulness groups." *Ryan M. Niemiec, PsyD, psychologist and author of* Mindfulness and Character Strengths: A Practical Guide to Flourishing, *education director of the VIA Institute on Character*

Building Competence in Mindfulness-Based Cognitive Therapy

Transcripts and Insights for Working With Stress, Anxiety, Depression, and Other Problems

Richard W. Sears
Foreword by Zindel V. Segal

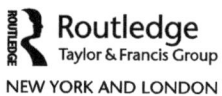

NEW YORK AND LONDON

First published 2015
by Routledge
711 Third Avenue, New York, NY 10017

and by Routledge
27 Church Road, Hove, East Sussex BN3 2FA

Routledge is an imprint of the Taylor & Francis Group, an informa business

© 2015 Richard W. Sears

The right of Richard W. Sears to be identified as author of this work has been asserted by him in accordance with sections 77 and 78 of the Copyright, Designs and Patents Act 1988.

All rights reserved. No part of this book may be reprinted or reproduced or utilised in any form or by any electronic, mechanical, or other means, now known or hereafter invented, including photocopying and recording, or in any information storage or retrieval system, without permission in writing from the publishers.

Trademark notice: Product or corporate names may be trademarks or registered trademarks, and are used only for identification and explanation without intent to infringe.

Library of Congress Cataloging in Publication Data
    Sears, Richard W., 1969–
Building competence in mindfulness-based cognitive therapy : transcripts and insights for working with stress, anxiety, depression, and other problems / by Richard W. Sears. — 1 Edition.
        pages cm
    Includes bibliographical references and index.
    1. Mindfulness-based cognitive therapy.   I. Title.
    RC489.M55S42 2015
    616.89'1425—dc23
    2014033639

ISBN: 978-0-415-85724-6 (hbk)
ISBN: 978-0-415-85725-3 (pbk)
ISBN: 978-0-203-79829-4 (ebk)

Typeset in Bembo
by Apex CoVantage, LLC

To Carrie Mason-Sears, for her many years of love and support

Contents

Illustrations	xi
Foreword by Zindel V. Segal	xii
Acknowledgments	xiv
1 Introduction	1

PART I
Building Competence · 9

2 Personal and Professional Competence	11
3 Building Competence in the Methods	23

PART II
Session Transcripts · 43

4 The Initial Session	45
5 Session 1: Awareness and Autopilot	63
6 Session 2: Living in Our Heads	79
7 Session 3: Gathering the Scattered Mind	97
8 Session 4: Recognizing Aversion	116
9 Session 5: Allowing/Letting Be	131
10 Session 6: Thoughts Are Not Facts	145
11 Session 7: Taking Care of Myself	161

12 Session 8: Extending New Learning   175

References   187
Index   195
About the Author   198

Illustrations

4.1	Stress curve	48
5.1	Raisin exercise	68
10.1	Tibetan bells	146
12.1	Graduation certificate	180
12.2	Rock exercise	184

All illustrations courtesy of Richard W. Sears

Foreword

At a meeting in Cambridge in 2000, John Teasdale, Mark Williams, and I were drafting the outline for the first edition of the mindfulness-based cognitive therapy treatment manual. We were confident with the empirical rationale that our book provided for combining the practice of mindfulness meditation with the tools of cognitive therapy but recognized that the clinical application of this approach might be challenging to therapists, as the training requirements were somewhat unorthodox at the time. In particular, in order to lead MBCT groups, we stated that it was necessary for the instructor to have a personal mindfulness practice and that familiarity with yoga, mindful movement, and experience running groups was also required. Placing personal preconditions ahead of the clinical implementation of an intervention was certainly not the standard approach to learning a manualized evidence-based treatment. Frankly, we worried that by asking for this dual skill set, we were restricting the potential pool of interested therapists, thereby preventing MBCT from achieving liftoff in spite of its promising clinical outcomes.

Our response to this dilemma was to do our best through both published and professional training resources in supporting instructors who offered the program. We ensured that the MBCT treatment manual provided concrete guidance regarding both the content and process of the eight group sessions, along with curricula, transcripts, troubleshooting tips, and patient handouts. We also committed to training MBCT instructors in a hybrid format that combined the features of a clinical workshop with a meditation retreat. We saw this as the best way to develop and build capacity in the dual skill set we considered essential.

Those following the field will undoubtedly recognize the changes that have occurred since 2000, especially how much more common it is for therapists to have some form of personal contemplative practice, be it meditation, yoga, or prayer, and the increasing number of clinical models available for bringing these views of the mind and its perturbations into patient care. Indeed, it is now possible to download numerous books, videos, and audio recordings of mindfulness practices. This is a welcome evolution, and yet amid this bounty, the need for careful training in MBCT persists. This is because MBCT was never intended for getting patients to simply practice meditation. Mindfulness, as is now recognized, offers access to mind states that are orthogonal to the habitual ruminative and aversion-oriented responding that is frequently triggered by negative affect. The systematic practice of mindfulness helps patients develop a different relationship to distressing emotions and, when combined with the cognitive-behavioral therapy (CBT) elements of the program, allow these skills to be increasingly available in everyday life.

Richard Sears has written a book that responds to this very need. The basic premise of the book is sound and timely—help MBCT therapists build competence by reading/observing the transcripts of real sessions. It is evocative, grounded, rich in detail, and skillful in laying out what actually happens in the eight sessions of MBCT. I don't know whether you have ever had the experience of sitting courtside or behind home plate at a basketball or baseball game, but that same quality of noticing all the detail and nuance in the game is available in much the same way in this book. By exposing his own work through transcripts, nuts-and-bolts guidance, and discussion, he has provided the reader with a special vantage point—you've got a front-row seat in his class and don't have to watch the group from farther away. Whether you are leading mindfulness practices, embodying presence and kindness in interactions with group members, or guiding inquiry, this book fills a significant void in the literature by supporting the ongoing professional development of MBCT instructors regardless of their novice, intermediate, or expert status. In just this way, *Building Competence in Mindfulness-Based Cognitive Therapy* extends the thread of our original discussions in 2000 and ensures a collective commitment to providing the best possible support and accompaniment to those who choose to undertake this work.

Zindel V. Segal, Ph.D.
Distinguished Professor of Psychology in Mood Disorders
University of Toronto Scarborough
Toronto, June 2014

Acknowledgments

Developing a new intervention that provides fresh perspectives and practical tools for effectively dealing with long-standing problems takes creativity, courage, and patience, often in the face of significant resistance from those invested in the way they have always done things. I deeply appreciate and salute Zindel Segal, Mark Williams, and John Teasdale for their tireless efforts to develop, test, and so freely share MBCT, as well as Jon Kabat-Zinn, Saki Santorelli, and Elana Rosenbaum, pioneers of mindfulness-based stress reduction (MBSR). I am especially honored that Dr. Segal took the time to write the foreword to this book.

It is wonderful how those I have met and worked with in the mindfulness community immediately feel like family. I am grateful for the friendship and inspiration of my MBCT colleagues and mentors: Dennis Tirch, Robert Denton, Susan Woods, Randye Semple, Jean Kristeller, Ryan Niemiec, Susan Albers, Sarah Bowen, Ruth Baer, and Mark Lau. I have a special feeling of gratitude for Alan Marlatt, who wrote an endorsement for my first mindfulness book only months before he passed away.

Many thanks to Anna Moore, senior editor at Routledge Mental Health, for approaching me and supporting me in bringing this volume into being. I am also very appreciative of Aarin Cox, Ashlyn Sears, and Kristy Donley for their diligent transcription work, and of Diane Baumer for her editing.

I am very thankful for the love and support of my family, Carrie Mason-Sears, Ashlyn Sears, Caylee Sears, Jeremy Rogers, Olivia and Brittney Taylor, Charles and Elfriede Sears, Brad Mason, and Linda and John Coghill.

I would like to express profound appreciation to Stephen K. Hayes for 30 years of mentorship, growth, and friendship, and to Paul Wonji Lynch for giving so freely of himself and helping me to see things in the moment just as they are.

I've been honored to work with a talented team of clinicians and mindfulness researchers: Sian Cotton, Melissa DelBello, Jeffery Strawn, Stefanie Stevenson, Nina McCune, and Rachel Wasson at the University of Cincinnati Center for Integrative Health & Wellness, UC College of Medicine, and Cincinnati Children's Hospital, as well as Kate Chard, Kristen Walter, and Lindsey Davidson at the Cincinnati VA.

A very heartfelt thanks to Steve and Sandi Amoils for their personal and professional support as well as to Nancy Merrell and all of the staff at Alliance Integrative Medicine for facilitating the opportunity to conduct so many MBCT groups in their agency, including the one transcribed here.

I am also appreciative of the growth-stimulating, postgroup discussions I have had over the years with my doctoral students and other professionals, especially Tina Luberto, Kristen Kraemer, Michelle Durling, Lauren Stahl, Julie Sell-Smith, James Foster, Tim Brannigan, Joe Behler, Kathy Schulz, Karen Byerly-Lamm, Cathy Giovanetti, Dean Gardner, and Claire Dean.

Most importantly, I am honored and grateful for the five individuals in this group who freely gave their permission to have these sessions recorded and transcribed so that we all might grow from their struggles and transformations.

1 Introduction

Mindfulness-based cognitive therapy (MBCT), first developed by Segal, Williams, and Teasdale (2013), is an 8-week, evidence-based program that integrates training in mindfulness skills with cognitive-behavioral therapy (CBT) techniques for working with stress, anxiety, depression, and other problems. Mindfulness, or awareness of present-moment experience, is developed through exercises designed to strengthen attentional capacity.

Zindel Segal (2013) describes four ways mindfulness can be helpful for clients. First, it fosters awareness, which counters the "automatic pilot" mode we often fall into by bringing conscious attention to habitual patterns of thinking and reacting. Second, it helps clients come into their present-moment experiences more often rather than getting stuck in past memories and future anticipations. Third, it develops more choicefulness, that is, it fosters response flexibility, allowing clients to become more aware of the choices they have in any given moment. Fourth, mindfulness practice improves affect tolerance, which helps clients to allow their feelings to rise and fall naturally rather than struggling with them or avoiding them through maladaptive behaviors.

Interventions utilizing mindfulness are continuing to gain attention due to the effectiveness demonstrated in clinical research. On the website of Division 12 (Society of Clinical Psychology) of the American Psychological Association (www.psychologicaltreatments.org), dialectical behavior therapy and acceptance and commitment therapy, both of which have a major mindfulness component, are listed as having "modest to strong research support," the same rating given to behavior therapy and cognitive-behavioral therapy. MBCT is listed under Cognitive Therapy for Depression, which is described as having "strong research support." MBCT and mindfulness-based stress reduction (MBSR) are also listed and reviewed in detail on the Substance Abuse and Mental Health Services Administration's National Registry of Evidence-Based Programs and Practices in the United States (www.nrepp.samhsa.gov). MBCT is also recommended for depression by the UK's National Institute for Health and Care Excellence (www.nice.org.uk).

Another reason mindfulness is gaining so much attention is due to the plethora of brain imaging studies demonstrating concrete changes in structure and functioning, even after 8 weeks of mindfulness practice, in both adults and children (e.g., Cotton, Luberto, Stahl, Sears, & DelBello, 2014; Davidson, Kabat-Zinn, Schumacher, Rosenkranz, Muller, et al., 2003; Farb, Segal, & Anderson, 2013; Farb, Segal, Mayberg, Bean, McKeon, & Anderson, 2007; Hölzel, Lazar, Gard, Schuman-Olivier, Vago, & Ott, 2011; Lazar, Kerr, Wasserman, Gray, Greve, et al., 2005; Siegel, 2007).

Clinicians are also becoming increasingly interested in mindfulness for their own self-care and clinical training (e.g., Davis & Hayes, 2011; Fulton, 2005; Shapiro, Brown, & Biegel, 2007). Interestingly, the clients of therapists who practice mindfulness have been shown to have better outcomes (Grepmair, Mietterlehner, Loew, Bachler, Rother, & Nickel, 2007).

The story of how MBCT came into being is described in the treatment manual (Segal, Williams, & Teasdale, 2013). Initially, the developers of MBCT, Zindel Segal, Mark Williams, and John Teasdale, were working to develop an effective, efficient intervention to prevent relapses of depression. The chances of becoming clinically depressed yet again increase with each episode of depression, and after two episodes of depression, there is a 70% to 80% chance of recurrence (Keller, Lavori, Lewis, & Klerman, 1983; Kupfer, 1991).

Meta-analyses of more than 40 studies demonstrate that there is no difference in negative thinking patterns between those who were between episodes of depression and those who had never been depressed (Ingram, Atchley, & Segal, 2011). It turns out that it is not negative thinking but dips in mood that lead to depressive relapse. Those who have previously experienced major depressive disorder take longer to recover from ordinary dips in mood. During this time, they are more vulnerable to reactivation of negative thinking, attitudes, and beliefs, leading to withdrawal behaviors and reduced activity levels, which can result in a downward mood spiral (Segal, Gemar, & Williams, 1999). This understanding led to a search for a new approach to preventing depression, and after consultation with Marsha Linehan, developer of dialectical behavior therapy (Linehan, 1993), and Jon Kabat-Zinn and colleagues, who developed mindfulness-based stress reduction (Kabat-Zinn, 2013), MBCT was born.

MBCT has been studied with rigorous, well-controlled clinical research, demonstrating significant reductions in depressive relapse rates, especially for those who have suffered three or more previous major depressive episodes (Hofmann, Sawyer, Witt, & Oh, 2010; Kuyken, Crane, & Dalgleish, 2012; Ma & Teasdale, 2004; Piet & Hougaard, 2011; Segal, Teasdale, & Williams, 2004; Teasdale, Segal, & Williams, 1995; Teasdale, Segal, Williams, Ridgeway, Soulsby, & Lau, 2000; Williams & Kuyken, 2012). MBCT has also been shown to be as effective as maintenance antidepressant pharmacotherapy (Kuyken, Byford, Byng, Dalgleish, Lewis, et al., 2010; Segal, Bieling, Young, MacQueen, Cooke, et al., 2010).

How Does MBCT Differ From Traditional CBT?

MBCT incorporates many cognitive-behavioral therapy (CBT) principles and techniques for working with thoughts, emotions, body sensations, and behaviors. The difference is in how clients are taught to relate to those aspects of themselves. Basically, what appears to be implicit in CBT is made explicit in MBCT.

For example, CBT methods often target change in the content of a client's cognitions, using systematic techniques to question the logic, utility, or validity of the thinking. A CBT therapist might teach a client to notice a negative automatic thought and to question the evidence for and against that thought. Clients can then train to restructure their thinking into a more rational or functional alternative (Sears, Tirch, & Denton, 2011). However, sometimes clients get into arguments in their own minds, because it is difficult to outthink oneself. Also, according to the principle of mood state-dependent memory, when one is depressed, the brain will have much easier access to depression-related memories (Segal & Lau, 2013; Ucros, 1989). For example, when a client becomes aware of a thought such as, "I can't do anything right," the client then asks, "What's the evidence?" The client may then respond with something like, "Well, I failed at school, work, and marriage." "But your partner had a part in the failed relationship." "But I'm the idiot who picked her." "What about getting your college degree?" "That's only because the instructors went easy on me." And so it can continue, *ad absurdum*.

Decades ago, Hollon and Beck (1986) acknowledged that change in cognitive content may not actually be the active ingredient in cognitive therapy. Subsequent component analyses have not proven that the cognitive challenging component actually adds value to the therapeutic effectiveness of CBT interventions (Longmore & Worrell, 2007; Sears, Tirch, & Denton, 2011). It appears that noticing, writing down, and challenging thoughts actually serves to foster a process known as "decentering" (Segal, Williams, & Teasdale, 2013).

In MBCT, clients are explicitly taught to practice this decentering from thought content, effectively changing their relationship to the thoughts, uncoupling them from their affective components. Clients learn to recognize that they *have* thoughts, emotions, and sensations instead of overly identifying with them (being in the center of them). In other words, when a thought arises like, "I can't do anything right," clients practice noticing, "I am having a thought that I can't do anything right." Instead of engaging in internal debates with intense thoughts, clients see them as possible signs of underlying emotional states such as stress, depression, or anxiety. Clients can then shift their attention from the thoughts to explore their present-moment emotions and body sensations. This awareness opens up more opportunity for conscious responding, such as allowing the underlying feelings to pass instead of fueling them with more struggle, taking some considered action to deal with the situation, actively engaging in self-care to address the anxiety or depression, or even going back to thinking if they so choose. Conscious responding prevents the client from automatically engaging in reactions, such as avoidance and withdrawal, that might worsen their symptoms.

As will be seen in the session transcripts, MBCT incorporates a number of CBT principles and techniques, such as the ABC model (that thoughts, feelings, and behaviors affect each other), thought records, recognition of automatic and maladaptive thought patterns (catastrophizing, generalizing, mind reading, all-or-nothing thinking, etc.), and relapse prevention plans. The main difference is that MBCT emphasizes a decentered, curious approach to noticing and questioning troublesome thoughts, then choosing what to do next rather than getting caught up in debating with those thoughts. Mindfulness skills, which strengthen attentional capacity, are the vehicle for systematically developing and reliably engaging this ability to notice automatic patterns and to relate differently to challenging experiences.

Varieties of MBCT

In the wake of its success with preventing depressive relapse, MBCT is now being studied and adapted for a variety of populations and presenting issues, such as addictions (Bowen, Chalwa, & Marlatt, 2010), bipolar disorder (Deckersbach, Hölzel, Eisner, Lazar, & Nierenberg, 2014), cancer (Bartley, 2011), children and adolescents (Semple & Lee, 2011), eating disorders (Kristeller & Wolever, 2011), health anxiety (Surawy, McManus, Muse, & Williams, 2014; Williams, McManus, Muse, & Williams, 2011), posttraumatic stress disorder (Sears & Chard, 2015), and tinnitus (Sadlier, Stephens, & Kennedy, 2008).

Seeing the variety of conditions helped by MBCT and by mindfulness in general reminds one of the fantastic claims made by charlatans selling elixirs. However, through the development of more awareness of one's present-moment experiences (however difficult), one can make better choices to more flexibly relate to a wide variety of life situations.

The program I present in this book is an MBCT program open to the general public, with the premise that an educational, skill-building mindfulness group will reduce stress and increase awareness, thereby helping a variety of conditions. Discussions of depression, anxiety, chronic pain, and other problems come up throughout the course or as needed based upon the particular group members. The anonymous evaluations given to participants at the end of these groups have shown that they are very important and helpful. I am currently collecting more controlled and detailed research on this approach, including data collected as part of Karen Byerly-Lamm's doctoral dissertation.

The Need for and Purpose of This Book

While each variation of the MBCT model requires specialized training, the core components of each are the development of mindfulness skills and the teaching of CBT principles. Though the delivery methods may be refined over time, the essential skills of mindfulness have been taught for thousands of years, and this natural human state of being is timeless and already present in each client. This book therefore serves as a general guide for developing the qualities of an MBCT instructor, facilitating the process of learning the variations of MBCT delivery.

MBCT is different from other types of interventions that mental health professionals are typically trained to do. This is not something one can learn simply as academic knowledge, and it is not an intervention done "to" the client. It is crucial for the clinician to experience, practice, and embody the core skills and principles of mindfulness. Rather than engaging the participants as if they were individual therapy clients to whom one is applying the techniques of cognitive-behavioral therapy, the facilitator models mindfulness in responding to present-moment experiences in the group. This is difficult for a beginner to understand without observing examples of how this is done. Unfortunately, because so few people are well trained in MBCT, there are often not enough groups close to where one lives to provide the opportunity to experience how these processes unfold over the course of 8 weeks.

The purpose of this book is to provide glimpses of what it might be like to take a group through all eight sessions of this experiential approach through exploring important considerations and through actual transcripts. Of course, every group is a little different, just as every individual psychotherapy session is different. The goal is not to imitate my style or to make your sessions like mine but to provide a sense of the attitudes and processes that are so crucial to making MBCT work effectively.

This book is for you, the clinician. We will not go into detail about definitions and theories of mindfulness, though the transcripts contain much of that. The resource list in the next chapter offers a number of suggestions for getting more background knowledge if you are not already familiar with mindfulness and its clinical applications. Because the entire MBCT curriculum, as well as details about its evidence base, can be found in other books, the emphasis here will be on the processes involved in implementation.

Readers who are serious about learning how to implement MBCT interventions will of course need to obtain the treatment protocol manual (Segal, Williams, & Teasdale, 2013), which provides detailed instructions for how to conduct each session, as well as access to audio recordings and handouts for participants. However, this volume can also serve as an introduction to MBCT. The best way to learn, as in any treatment modality, is to experience it for oneself. Reading through the conversations and exercises in this book can give one a feel for what MBCT is all about, and if the reader chooses to learn more, the concepts in the treatment manuals will likely make more sense.

The next chapter will set the foundation by describing how to build personal and professional competence in MBCT. The chapter will describe the essential qualifications and training needed to become a competent facilitator, provide a list of resources for further study, and discuss the importance of the therapist's own personal mindfulness practice.

The third chapter will explore important considerations for the competent delivery of the MBCT protocol. The focus will be on processes, such as how to lead the mindfulness exercises and the crucial phase of inquiry that follows. The chapter will also explore issues related to working with challenging clients, considerations for training and supervising students, and the practical issues of running an MBCT group.

The bulk of this book consists of actual transcripts of an 8-week MBCT group. Each chapter begins with a description of the important concepts of the session, followed by a transcript of the entire session with clients' questions, comments, and reactions.

The participants in these transcripts are real people, though all identifying information has been removed or changed. They all freely gave their permission to record the sessions. Originally, I recorded several groups and considered combining them into a sort of composite for teaching purposes, but I felt that following the same individuals gives the reader a better sense of the growth process that happens. This group was smaller than usual, having only five members, resulting in a more casual, more intimate feel than is typical for a larger group.

The transcripts have undergone some minor editing to make them smoother and more natural to read. Unfortunately, listening to the recordings as I compare them to the transcripts, the words on the page seem terribly flat. The reader will miss the tone, emphases, silences, body language, aliveness, and dynamics of being present in an actual group. It is also difficult to sense the warmth and acceptance that I am modeling.

Because the mindfulness exercises take up a large part of each session and are already transcribed in the protocol books, they have been edited out to save space. One can find free recordings of the exercises on the Internet, including my own website, www.psych-insights.com. The groups are not simply a place to read transcripts of exercises, which participants can get from listening to CDs. The essential ingredient of an MBCT group is the inquiry and processing that takes place when the participants are learning to internalize the principles of mindfulness and how to integrate them into their daily lives.

Though small talk naturally emerges from an atmosphere that is warm and inviting, I have cut most of this out to save space. There are also places where we do not strictly follow the formal curriculum. For empirical studies, careful adherence to reproducible protocols is very important. For ongoing clinical work, minor adjustments for the particular group, modeling flexibility and present-moment experiencing, can be priceless. While you will find all of the elements of the protocol covered in each group, you will also find natural digressions to material relevant for the individuals in this group. However, even when the session gets "off track" in terms of content, the principles of mindfulness are still being followed, because the facilitator is joining into the developing mindfulness processes of the participants rather than automatically squelching the process artificially to rigidly adhere to content structure at every moment.

Of note, this group was conducted before the second edition of the MBCT manual was published. You may notice a few minor differences in protocol here, such as viewing the *Healing From Within* video, but the general format is the same.

Even in the couple of years since this was recorded, I feel that I have grown and matured as an MBCT therapist, and I endeavor to continue to do so. The participants and graduate students attending each group never fail to share and inspire new insights. I considered starting a newer set of recordings, but perhaps this will serve as a reminder to engage with reality as it is and to let go of the desire for some kind of perfection in the delivery of the group.

In each MBCT session, we open with a mindfulness exercise, which models starting with this moment before addressing challenges (Segal, 2008). Similarly, this book will start with building personal and professional competence before getting into the details of conducting MBCT groups. However, if you are relatively new to MBCT, you might choose to skip down to the actual transcripts of the groups, ideally downloading and practicing the mindfulness exercises as well, and then come back to the earlier chapters. This may provide a better understanding of the material covered in the groups and how it might be presented to clients, giving context to the suggestions and considerations in the next two chapters.

The good news is that you do not have to memorize everything you read about mindfulness. The concepts in the manuals are very important, and I hope this book will open up new perspectives and deepen your understanding, but the bottom line is that the best way to learn is through your own practice. Of course, having your own regular practice will take a strong commitment to yourself and to the people you serve. Are you ready to begin?

Part I
Building Competence

2 Personal and Professional Competence

Although mindfulness is a natural human process that we all possess already, people often come to MBCT groups because they are suffering from serious life problems. Therefore, if you wish to lead these groups, you must possess the appropriate professional qualifications, receive training to develop the necessary knowledge, skills, and attitudes, and establish a personal mindfulness practice.

Currently, there is no universally recognized, mandatory certification process to use MBCT, and there likely never will be. Most licensing boards and ethics codes basically state that "you are competent to do what you are competent to do." However, if one is challenged, licensing boards may inquire into current, reasonable standards of competency based on the best practices of peers who work with the particular population and intervention in question.

For some specialties, there are clearly defined guidelines, such as the guidelines for child custody evaluations established by the American Psychological Association (2010). Neuropsychologists typically expect those who use the title to have completed a 2-year postdoctoral training in the specialty.

Many areas of mental health practice, such as cognitive behavioral therapy, have training institutes, certification programs, and board certification processes, which provide solid credentials to document that one has received the necessary training. Likewise, there are some wonderful training programs available to those who would like to learn MBCT, such as MBSR Teacher Certification through the Oasis Institute at the UMass Center for Mindfulness, the applied MBCT facilitation certificate program at the University of Toronto, and the Master of Studies degree in MBCT at the University of Oxford, UK.

Though training programs such as those listed are ideal, most practitioners of psychological interventions, like CBT, psychodynamic, humanistic, and MBCT, are not formally credentialed due to the often enormous time, money, and travel commitments involved. So how do you demonstrate competence? By building a case that you have received sufficient training based on such things as graduate school education, supervised experience, seminars, books, and professional consultation, in line with the recommendations of experts in the particular modality.

Following are suggestions to build competence in MBCT based on generally accepted standards (Crane, 2009; Crane, Kuyken, Williams, Hastings, Cooper, & Fennell, 2012; Segal, Williams, & Teasdale, 2013; UK Network for Mindfulness-Based Teacher Training Organisations, 2011; Woods, 2014).

Basic Qualifications

Licensure as a Mental Health Professional

One of the predecessors of MBCT, mindfulness-based stress reduction (MBSR), was developed to be delivered by competent instructors, but professional licensure is not necessary. However, due to the clinical nature of the presenting issues in most MBCT groups, it is important to be licensed in your jurisdiction to provide mental health services. Even though MBCT is considered more of a psychoeducational, skill-building group rather than a traditional group psychotherapy intervention (Coelho, Canter, & Ernst, 2007; Williams, McManus, Muse, & Williams, 2011), clinical knowledge and skills are needed to understand the nature of the struggles the clients are facing and to handle any unexpected mental health issues that arise. When using MBCT for individual work, it is important to clarify up front what the expectations are, and it is usually best to treat the sessions as psychotherapy.

Of course, if you are a licensed mental health professional, you are held to the standards, ethical guidelines, and regulations of your profession, even for an educational group. Years ago, I was giving a workshop to psychologists on consultation and coaching, and someone asked if you were a licensed psychologist but called yourself a coach, if you were held to the standards of a psychologist. Someone from our state ethics committee was in the audience and did some research. Basically, the answer is yes. While you might call yourself a psychologist in one setting and a coach in another, you are a licensed psychologist regardless of what you call yourself, so you are answerable to any complaints filed with the State Board.

Generalist Knowledge

When group participants come, they are often struggling with a variety of life stressors, and many have mental health diagnoses. When they are finally asked to sit with their experiences and explore them, a variety of issues can come up. Therefore, an MBCT facilitator must have the breadth of clinical training to understand and feel comfortable working with a variety of conditions, such as anxiety, panic, depression, trauma, and suicidal ideation.

Competence in Working With Diverse Populations

In the early days of psychology and psychiatry, the major influencers were white males. As Robert Guthrie (2003) so poignantly stated in the title of his book on the history of psychology, *Even the Rat Was White*. The critical importance of acquiring and maintaining competence in working with diverse populations has been increasingly recognized in recent decades, as reflected in the ethics codes and practice guidelines of organizations such as the American Psychological Association (APA, 2002, 2003; Ponterotto, Casas, Suzuki, & Alexander, 2010). Licensing boards have sanctioned clinicians who did not work competently with diverse clients.

Although there were some significant exceptions (e.g., Hayes, 2007; Ting-Toomey, 2009; Vacarr, 2001), there has been a dearth of research investigating diversity variables in mindfulness-based interventions, though this important topic has gained more attention in recent years (e.g., Masuda, 2014; Sears, Tirch, & Denton, 2011; Woidneck, Pratt, Gundy, Nelson, & Twohig, 2012). Mindfulness- and acceptance-based therapies appear to be helpful for diverse populations, though it is important for the clinician to be sensitive to diversity issues in the delivery of these interventions (Fuchs, Lee, Roemer, & Orsillo, 2013).

Since mindfulness is about noticing, MBCT facilitators should be conscious of and comfortable with skillfully handling issues of diversity that arise within the group, such as microaggressions (Sue et al., 2007). For example, for a member of the dominant culture to say something like "I don't see color" implies that the values and heritage of those of a different background are not important (Helms, 1992). Though it need not become the focus of the group, ignoring a discriminatory comment is a subtle form of condoning it.

Moving beyond an understanding of individual and cultural differences, social justice factors are also important to keep in mind (Fouad, Gerstein, & Toporek, 2006). Social justice involves awareness of the inequities in power and opportunity that still exist in society today and calls on those of us with power and influence to be change makers to foster a more fair and tolerant world. For example, clinicians must be careful not to make assumptions about things like access to resources and comfort with technology and should consider offering scholarships for the groups and loaning out CD players. Other factors, such as the degree to which clients value individualism versus collectivism, will play a role in discussions of self-care. Since mindfulness increases awareness, clients may find themselves more aware of discrimination and its impact upon them. MBCT clinicians have a wonderful opportunity to have an open dialogue about what acceptance means in such circumstances and must be careful not to dismiss legitimate concerns, to imply that it is "all in their heads," or to encourage action that could make the situation worse.

It can be very difficult at times to openly discuss matters of diversity, because we open ourselves up to potential conflict and to the possibility that we will discover that we still hold on to our own subtle biases. As with mindfulness, competence in this area requires us to do our own work (Sears, Tirch, & Denton, 2011).

14   *Part I: Building Competence*

Working Knowledge of Cognitive-Behavioral Therapy

Since MBCT builds on CBT principles, it is important to have training in the principles of classical and operant conditioning, behavioral techniques, and cognitive therapy. Countless workshops and online trainings are now available, and several books are listed in the resources section of this chapter for those who need a refresher.

Working Knowledge of Group Dynamics and Interventions

Even though MBCT is conducted more as a class than as a group intervention, the group is a significantly beneficial factor in MBCT (Allen, Bromley, Kuyken, & Sonnenberg, 2009; Finucane & Mercer, 2006; Mason & Hargreaves, 2001; Smith, Graham, & Senthinathan, 2007; Williams, McManus, Muse, & Williams, 2011). Therefore, a working knowledge of group processes is important for such things as maintaining group cohesiveness, keeping the group on task, and skillfully working with challenging clients with techniques like shifting between content and process (Corey, 2012; Yalom & Leszcz, 2005). From this knowledge base, training and experience in how the MBCT approach differs from an interpersonal learning type of group is important. This will be discussed further in the next chapter.

Content-Related Expertise

Depending on the nature of the group, the clinician will also need content-specific expertise in addition to learning the nuances of the specific MBCT-based protocol. When using the original MBCT protocol to prevent depressive relapse (Segal, Williams, & Teasdale, 2013), it is important to have a working knowledge of such things as the nature and symptoms of depression, Beck's (1967) cognitive triad, and the factors that lead to relapse. Mindfulness-based relapse prevention for addictive behaviors (MBRP: Bowen, Chawla, & Marlatt, 2010) requires competence in addictions work and motivational interviewing skills. MBCT for children (MBCT-C: Semple & Lee, 2011) requires comfort in working with children and adolescents, the ability to discuss concepts using developmentally appropriate language, and a working knowledge of the adaptions of the exercises to be shorter, more concrete, more active, and more engaging of the senses.

Some populations may require significant adaptions and clinician expertise. In PTSD, the traumatic event was so horrible that the client does not want to remember it, but the brain sends powerful messages that this event is important to learn from for future survival. The flooding of glucocorticoids disrupts the ability of the hippocampus to lay down and retrieve coherent memories, resulting in seemingly random eruptions of thoughts and emotionally charged memories. Since one of the major dynamics of PTSD is struggling to avoid, asking someone to suddenly become mindful of their thoughts, emotions, and body sensations has to be done in a carefully controlled way (Sears & Chard, 2015). Mindfulness can be used as an adjunctive tool to traditional trauma exposure work, or the MBCT curriculum could be delivered to the client in individual sessions after completing an initial trauma treatment protocol such as cognitive processing therapy (Resick, Monson, & Chard, 2008) or prolonged exposure therapy (Foa, Hembree, & Rothbaum, 2007).

Ongoing Personal Mindfulness Practice

Unlike other interventions, it is crucial for MBCT instructors to personally practice what they are teaching to clients. We will discuss this in detail later in this chapter.

Training in MBCT Delivery

Assuming competence in the previously mentioned areas, the best way to learn MBCT is to experience it for yourself. Segal, Williams, and Teasdale (2013) recommend going through the entire 8-week course at least three times, once as a participant for your own learning, once as a trainee to pay attention to didactic methods, and once as a cotherapist to gain practice in facilitation.

Of course, you may not have easy access to a weekly MBCT group. Because it was first developed in the late 1970s, you are more likely to find an MBSR group by searching the directory of instructors at the UMass Center for Mindfulness (www.umassmed.edu/cfm). MBSR programs are great for learning mindfulness and for learning the inquiry process, but bear in mind that the program has a different emphasis than MBCT and may or may not be run by a mental health professional.

MBCT teacher training intensives, in which the entire curriculum is taught over the course of multiple days, are another option for those who are not able to attend the 8-week groups.

Online training programs can also be a helpful supplement for learning MBCT in a structured way. At the very least, you can take yourself through a self-paced program such as that offered in *The Mindful Way Workbook* (Teasdale, Williams, & Segal, 2014).

Once you are ready to begin leading your own groups, it will be important to have supervision or at least professional consultation from more experienced MBCT trainers. Ideally, and with the participants' permission, you can audio record your sessions to get feedback on the mindful inquiry process, which is the most subtle skill for MBCT facilitators to learn.

The next section lists a variety of books, videos, and audio recordings to build your MBCT knowledge base.

Resources

MBCT Curriculum Books

Segal, Z., Williams, M., & Teasdale, J. (2013). *Mindfulness-based cognitive therapy for depression* (2nd ed.). New York: Guilford Press.

Teasdale, J., Williams, M., & Segal, Z. (2014). *The mindful way workbook: An 8-week program to free yourself from depression and emotional distress.* New York: Guilford Press.

Williams, M., Teasdale, J., Segal, Z., & Kabat-Zinn, J. (2007). *The mindful way through depression: Freeing yourself from chronic unhappiness.* New York: Guilford Press.

MBCT-Related Books and Articles

Bartley, T. (2011). *Mindfulness-based cognitive therapy for cancer.* London, UK: Wiley-Blackwell.

Bowen, S., Chawla, N., & Marlatt, A. (2010). *Mindfulness-based relapse prevention for addictive behaviors: A clinician's guide.* New York: Guilford Press.

Collard, P. (2013). *Mindfulness-based cognitive therapy for dummies.* Chichester, West Sussex, UK: John Wiley & Sons.

Crane, R. (2009). *Mindfulness-based cognitive therapy.* London and New York: Routledge.

Crane, R., Kuyken, W., Williams, M., Hastings, R., Cooper, L., & Fennell, M. (2012). Competence in teaching mindfulness-based courses: Concepts, development, and assessment. *Mindfulness, 3,* 76–84. DOI: 0.1007/s12671-011-0073-2

Deckersbach, T., Hölzel, B., Eisner, L., Lazar, S., & Nierenberg, A. (2014). *Mindfulness-based cognitive therapy for bipolar disorder.* New York: Guilford Press.

Sears, R. (2014). *Mindfulness: Living through challenges and enriching your life in this moment.* London, UK: Wiley-Blackwell.

Sears, R., & Chard, K. (2015). *Mindfulness-based cognitive therapy for posttraumatic stress disorder.* London, UK: Wiley-Blackwell.

Sears, R., Tirch, D., & Denton, R. (2011). *Mindfulness in clinical practice.* Sarasota, FL: Professional Resource Press.

Segal, Z., Teasdale, J., Williams, M., & Gemar, M. (2002). The mindfulness-based cognitive therapy adherence scale: Inter-rater reliability, adherence to protocol and treatment distinctiveness. *Clinical Psychology & Psychotherapy, 9*(2), 131–138. DOI: 10.1002/cpp.320

Semple, R., & Lee, J. (2011). *Mindfulness-based cognitive therapy for anxious children.* Oakland, CA: New Harbinger Publications, Inc.

Williams, M., & Penman, D. (2011). *Mindfulness: An eight-week plan for finding peace in a frantic world.* Emmaus, PA: Rodale Books.

Woods, S. (2013). Building a framework for mindful inquiry. www.slwoods.com

Other Relevant Mindfulness Books and Articles

Albers, S. (2003). *Eating mindfully: How to end mindless eating and enjoy a balanced relationship with food.* Oakland, CA: New Harbinger Publications, Inc.

Bögels, S., & Restifo, K. (2014). *Mindful parenting: A guide for mental health practitioners.* New York: Springer.

Didonna, F. (Ed.). (2009). *Clinical handbook of mindfulness.* New York: Springer.

Duncan, L., & Bardacke, N. (2010). Mindfulness-based childbirth and parenting education: Promoting family mindfulness during the perinatal period. *Journal of Child & Family Studies, 19,* 190–202. DOI: 10.1007/s10826-009-9313-7

Fulton, P. (2005). Mindfulness as clinical training. In C. Germer, R. Siegel, & P. Fulton (Eds.), *Mindfulness and psychotherapy*. New York: Guilford Press.

Gunaratana, H. (2011). *Mindfulness in plain English*. Boston: Wisdom Publications.

Hölzel, B., Lazar, S., Gard, T., Schuman-Olivier, Z., Vago, D., & Ott, U. (2011). How does mindfulness meditation work? Proposing mechanisms of action from a conceptual and neural perspective. *Perspectives on Psychological Science, 6*(6) 537–559. DOI: 10.1177/1745691611419671

Kabat-Zinn, J. (1994). *Wherever you go there you are*. New York: Hyperion.

Kabat-Zinn, J. (2006). *Coming to our senses: Healing ourselves and the world through mindfulness*. New York: Hyperion.

Kabat-Zinn, J. (2013). *Full catastrophe living: Using the wisdom of your body and mind to face stress, pain, and illness* (rev. ed.). New York: Bantam.

Kristeller, J., Baer, R., & Quillian, R. (2006). Mindfulness-based approaches to eating disorders. In R. A. Baer (Ed.), *Mindfulness and acceptance-based interventions: Conceptualization, application, and empirical support* (pp. 75–91). San Diego, CA: Elsevier.

Kristeller, J., & Wolever, R. (2011). Mindfulness-based eating awareness training for treating binge eating disorder: The conceptual foundation. *Eating Disorders, 19*(1), 49–61. DOI: 10.1080/10640266.2011.533605

Masuda, A. (2014). *Mindfulness and acceptance in multicultural competency: A contextual approach to sociocultural diversity in theory and practice*. Oakland, CA: New Harbinger Publications.

McBee, L. (2008). *Mindfulness-based elder care: A CAM model for frail elders and their caregivers*. New York: Springer Pub.

McCown, D., Reibel, D., & Micozzi, M. (2011). *Teaching mindfulness: A practical guide for clinicians and educators*. New York: Springer.

Niemiec, R. (2014). *Mindfulness and character strengths: A practical guide to flourishing*. Boston, MA: Hogrefe Publishing.

Santorelli, S. (2000). *Heal thy self: Lessons on mindfulness in medicine*. New York: Crown Publishers.

Siegel, D. (2007). *The mindful brain: Reflection and attunement in the cultivation of well-being*. New York: W. W. Norton & Company.

Other Relevant Clinical Books

Corey, G. (2012). *Theory & practice of group counseling* (8th ed.). Belmont, CA: Brooks/Cole, Cengage Learning.

Greenberger, D., & Padesky, C. (1995). *Mind over mood: A cognitive therapy treatment manual for clients*. New York: Guilford Press.

Leahy, R. (2003). *Cognitive therapy techniques: A practitioner's guide*. New York: Guilford Press.

McMullin, R. (2000). *The new handbook of cognitive therapy techniques* (rev. ed.). New York: W. W. Norton.

Miller, W., & Rollnick, S. (2013). *Motivational interviewing: Helping people change* (3rd ed.). New York: Guilford Press.

Ponterotto, J., Casas, J., Suzuki, L., & Alexander, C. (2010). *Handbook of multicultural counseling* (3rd ed.). Los Angeles, CA: SAGE Publications.

Sears, R., & Niblick, A. (Eds.). (2014). *Perspectives on religion and spirituality in psychotherapy*. Sarasota, FL: Professional Resource Press.

Yalom, I., & Leszcz, M. (2005). *The theory and practice of group psychotherapy* (5th ed.). New York: Basic Books.

Audio and Video Workshops

Kabat-Zinn, J., & Moyers, B. (1993). *Healing from within* [video]. New York: Ambrose Video. Episode of the Bill Moyers series, *Healing and the Mind*, that follows Jon Kabat-Zinn taking a group through the eight weeks of an MBSR course.

Sears, R. (2012). *Mindfulness-based cognitive therapy: An introduction and overview* [video file]. Washington, DC: American Psychological Association. http://apa.bizvision.com/product/2012-cew-recordings/mindfulnessbasedcognitivetherapyanintroductionandoverview(7552). Seven-hour on-demand CE video workshop.

Segal, Z. (2008). *Mindfulness-based cognitive therapy for depression and anxiety* [CD]. Lancaster, PA: J&K Seminars, LLC. Two-day MBCT workshop on audio.

Segal, Z., & Carlson, J. (2005). *Mindfulness-based cognitive therapy for depression* [DVD]. Washington, DC: American Psychological Association. www.apa.org/pubs/videos/4310714.aspx. DVD video of Zindel Segal conducting the first session of MBCT, with an interview with Jon Carlson.

Williams, M. (2009). *Mindfulness-based cognitive therapy and the prevention of depression: Training video*. New York: Association for Behavioral and Cognitive Therapies. DVD video of Mark Williams covering basic principles of MBCT.

Selected Websites

Mindfulness-based cognitive therapy
www.mbct.com

The Centre for Mindfulness Studies in Toronto
www.mindfulnessstudies.com

UCSD Center for Mindfulness, Mindfulness-Based Professional Training Institute
www.mbpti.org

The Center for Mindfulness in Medicine, Health Care, and Society, University of Massachusetts Medical School
www.umassmed.edu/cfm

Jon Kabat-Zinn's mindfulness audio recordings
www.mindfulnesscds.com

UK Network for Mindfulness-Based Teacher Training Organisations
mindfulnessteachersuk.org.uk

Mindfulness Research Guide
www.mindfulexperience.org

Mindful Awareness Research Center
marc.ucla.edu

Mindfulness-Based Relapse Prevention for Addictive Behaviors
www.mindfulrp.com

The Center for Mindful Eating
www.thecenterformindfuleating.org

Richard Sears (author's website)
www.psych-insights.com

Richard Davidson (brain research)
richardjdavidson.com

Susan Albers (mindful eating)
eatingmindfully.com

Susan Woods (MBSR/MBCT trainer)
www.slwoods.com

Your Own Personal Practice

The resources listed contain a wealth of information, but the real challenge is in integrating and embodying mindfulness in your daily life as well as in your clinical work. The best way to do that is through your own personal practice.

It would be disingenuous to talk to participants about the importance of practice if you are not doing it yourself. After all, no one would want a fitness trainer who never exercised, and it is easy to see if a trainer is out of shape. Interestingly, when I practice regularly, few people ask me if I do, but during times when I have been less consistent, I was asked more often. Also, when I practiced less regularly, my clients were less likely to do the homework themselves. Without words, something was being transmitted. The MBCT founders reported similar experiences as they began their work (Segal, Williams, & Teasdale, 2013).

It is wonderful to be able to practice mindfulness ourselves while we are leading groups. When I got busy for a period of time, and I was leading groups or clients in exercises throughout the day, I thought perhaps I did not also need to practice on my own. However, I noticed a big difference in how I felt when I resumed my personal practice. When we do individual psychotherapy all day long, we often experience personal growth, and yet we would never think of that as a replacement for our own therapy or self-development.

Having first learned mindfulness meditation 30 years ago, I have been through many ups and downs in terms of regularity of practice, from zealous eagerness to feeling like I had absolutely no need for "formal" practice. And yet, there is no doubt whatsoever that whenever I sit down to practice, I'm glad I did. Even when difficult thoughts and emotions are present, they tend to open up and settle, my mind becomes clearer, and I feel more present in the rest of my day.

So why is it so hard to do this regularly? As we discuss in the course, there are a number of reasons. As an instructor committed to sharing the benefits of mindfulness, it is important for us to experience the normal ups and downs that our clients will experience in establishing a regular practice. If it had always been easy for you to practice every day and you immediately went into a clear, blissful state of mind each time, you would be a terrible teacher. Most clients would not be able to relate to you, and you would have difficulty understanding their struggles. Having experience with our own practice helps us relate to all the normal challenges, obstacles, bizarre experiences, and delights that will come up for our clients.

So give yourself permission to experience all the challenges everyone else does, as described in the protocol manual (Segal, Williams, & Teasdale, 2013). It comes down to becoming aware of the challenges, watching the flow of thoughts about whether you should do it, exploring any sense of resistance that is present, and just making the choice to do it every day anyway. No matter what our past experiences have been, we simply start fresh, right now in this moment, which is really what mindfulness is all about.

As an added bonus, a regular mindfulness practice can be an important component of clinician self-care. Professional caregivers are often notoriously bad at taking care of themselves, because we are trained to attend to the needs of others (Barnett, 2007). In a survey by Pope and Tabachnick (1993), more than half of the clinicians reported that their concerns about clients impacted their personal functioning. Another survey revealed that almost 60% of practicing psychologists kept working even when they were too distressed to be effective (Pope, Tabachnick, & Keith-Spiegel, 1987).

Choiceless Awareness Practice

Zen teacher Wonji Dharma, quoting his teacher Seung Sahn, often says, "Zen practice is very simple. What do you see, hear, feel, smell, and taste, moment after moment after moment?" (Dharma, 2010, p. 9). This is an excellent description of the practice known as "choiceless awareness" (Kabat-Zinn, 2012; Krishnamurti, 2012).

Choiceless awareness is mindfulness of present-moment experiences without staying with any particular object of awareness. This practice is "advanced" due to its simplicity. It is typically only touched upon in the groups, but it is a wonderful daily practice, especially for MBCT leaders to foster their moment-to-moment contact with the experiences that unfold throughout the group sessions.

Through this practice, we recognize that there is just this moment. If I were standing in front of you right now, could you show me something that is not in the present moment? Even our thoughts and memories are happening right now. We experience the fact that no one moment is any better than any other moment, because other moments only exist in our minds right now. Experiencing this, our minds can more easily let go of the habitual stream of compulsive judgments and comparisons.

Although I might briefly introduce this practice to my MBCT groups, it often sounds a bit philosophical to those new to mindfulness, though in fact it is a very concrete experience. However, as a facilitator, demonstrating an embodiment of this principle in a natural, wordless, unforced way is extremely powerful.

This experience can be challenging to describe in words, which is why metaphors are often used, such as keeping a mind like a mirror. Reflections come and go and do not stick to the mirror. Likewise, this practice is about noticing our experiences from moment to moment. A sound is heard, then fades away. A thought arises, lingers, then passes away. Body sensations come and go. This skill is important to help MBCT instructors remain aware of the variety of experiences all the group members may be having as the session progresses while also keeping track of the time and the curriculum content.

Ultimately, the words you hear on the recordings of mindfulness exercises are meant to be a scaffold, a structure to help build your awareness. Eventually, words get in the way of direct experience. As long as you are always filtering your experience through words, you are prone to getting caught up in them, or you may become overly reliant on clever explanations. Though words are crucial for communicating and teaching, by experiencing your practice more directly, you will drop the need to remember the "right" words to describe something or the "correct" explanation. You will no longer have to imitate or remember the words of anyone else. Your practice will become more stable over time, allowing you to model a direct, genuine presence for clients in a natural way, not forced or put on. You will then more easily let go of the need to impress anyone or the fear of being exposed as a "fake" and be more fully yourself.

Maintaining Competence

Just as licensed mental health professionals need continuing-education credits to remain competent in their clinical work, it is important to maintain contact with others teaching MBCT and related interventions, to attend retreats and workshops with mindfulness teachers, and of course to keep up with your personal mindfulness practice.

Recently, I attended an all-day workshop with Zindel Segal and Mark Lau on MBCT. Randye Semple, the lead developer of MBCT-C, sat next to me in the front row. Before we started, Zindel smiled and said, "What are you doing here, Randye? You know all this stuff!" She smiled and said, "I like to keep a beginner's mind."

This is a key attitude of mindfulness. When we are isolated and lose our beginner's mind, there is a risk of "drift" over time and the possibility of getting lost in our own idiosyncrasies. We may end up confusing "this is the way I've always done it" with "this is the most effective way to do it." Sometimes those two are very different.

When I first started practicing as a young teenager, I would not have wanted to hear that you are never "done." But how could you possibly be "done" with the present moment? Every moment is new and fresh. It is only our thinking that tells us we already "know" what is happening in any given moment. We can remind ourselves to sort out thoughts ("I already know this stuff") and feelings (boredom) from the actual physical sensations we are experiencing moment to moment, which are always new and changing.

It is easy to attend to novel things, but it takes practice to cultivate wonder at daily, routine things. Even our mindfulness practice can become another conditioned response. After leading the same MBCT course over and over, eating hundreds of raisins and looking at hundreds of rocks, I jokingly tell colleagues, "I can do this mindfulness stuff in my sleep!" It is a very advanced skill to be mindful of mindfulness techniques, to be in the moment when teaching others how to be in the moment. If we fail to do this, we become parrots repeating good ideas and miss the nuances of each moment and each individual with whom we are interacting, and what we convey is no longer fresh or genuine.

Connecting with others who teach and practice mindfulness is important to keep us both inspired and grounded. Attending teacher training intensives and retreats and connecting with local meditation centers keeps us immersed in the practice.

With modern technology, it is also now possible to instantly download hundreds of books, videos, and mindfulness recordings. Once you have established your practice and have experienced the foundational training, you will recognize which ones will be helpful (many of them may have "mindfulness" in the title but are not actually teaching mindfulness). Readings and new recordings can help to keep you motivated and up-to-date on the latest research and your practice fresh. Exposure to other ways of expressing these ideas and conducting exercises will also broaden your ability to communicate and facilitate mindfulness for others.

3 Building Competence in the Methods

Once you gain experience with practicing mindfulness and the theoretical knowledge of how MBCT works, you are ready to begin learning methods for teaching these principles to the suffering clients who come to you seeking relief. Experiencing it for yourself is crucial, but we must also make the link to how it can be incorporated into our clinical work. Just because we have an experience for ourselves or have practiced for decades does not necessarily mean it will translate into something clinically useful for our clients (Segal, 2013).

Speaking Their Language

Due to the current popularity of mindfulness, some clients may seek you out knowing exactly what they are looking for after reading books about it or practicing some other form of meditation. However, most clients will be ordinary human beings seeking relief from their suffering. It is therefore crucial for clinicians to be able to put these concepts into practical language understandable to the particular clients with whom they are working. Many mindfulness practitioners have a passion for what they do, but clients are often just looking for concrete help. No matter how good the practice of mindfulness sounds, they will ask, "What is the goal of this, and how is this going to help me?" It is a fair question—that is why they are coming to you as a professional (Segal, 2013). They do not usually want you to tell them to practice for 40 years until eventually they get the paradox of non-doing. If clients do not "buy in," they will not join the group or will not practice and will not benefit much from the program.

Because mindfulness is often associated with spiritual groups, it is important to be clear that MBCT is a secular program. While I personally have a strong connection to traditional Zen, I keep it separate from my professional role as clinician for MBCT groups. I do not ring bells, wear beads, burn incense, or sit on the floor, because in my community, that would be seen as odd.

In my research with MBCT with veterans with posttraumatic stress disorder (PTSD) with Kate Chard (Sears & Chard, 2015), most subjects had never heard of mindfulness and would make reference to "hippies" and "tree hugging." Davis and Luedtke (2013), in their work using mindfulness-based cognitive-behavioral conjoint therapy for PTSD, have found that veterans are much more receptive to the terms "situational awareness" and "awareness training."

When I give continuing education workshops to other clinicians, I talk about how mindfulness relates to attentional pathways, emotional regulation, negative reinforcement, exposure therapy, and evidence-based practice. In organizational settings, I talk about burnout, employee turnover, lost productivity, and the bottom line (McConnell & Sears, 2014; Sears, Rudisill, & Mason-Sears, 2006; Sears, Tirch, & Denton, 2011; Williams, 2006). Peter Senge uses the term "presence" (Senge, Scharmer, Jaworski, & Flowers, 2004), and Daniel Goleman and Jon Kabat-Zinn (2007) talk about mindfulness as an aspect of emotional intelligence.

At the health care agencies where I do my groups, most participants come because they are hurting, anxious, or otherwise suffering and are just looking to try something new. They often come in solely on faith through a referral from their physician. You will see in the transcripts the language I use for these groups.

Leading the Mindfulness Exercises

A large portion of MBCT groups is spent guiding and then processing mindfulness exercises. The protocol manual contains all the scripts for the exercises (Segal, Williams, & Teasdale, 2013), and there are many good recordings from which to learn. Below are some considerations about the process itself.

Transitioning Into the Exercise

While we do not want to imply that there is a difference between a mindful state and "normal" consciousness, a little preparation signals that we are going to choose to pay more attention to our current experiences. I typically start by asking participants to sit in whatever way is comfortable for them and perhaps to get the "pre-fidgets" out of the way—stretching or moving around as needed to be comfortable. In early sessions, I mention that it is okay to move during the exercise so they are not concerned about that. I then ask them either to shade their eyes and look down at the floor or close their eyes. Early on, I mention that they can experiment to see which works best for them. If they are feeling sleepy, it is probably better to leave the eyes open a little. Those with a trauma history often feel uncomfortable keeping their eyes closed in a room full of strangers.

Before getting into the specific exercise, I often suggest they take a few moments to appreciate being able to sit still, since they may have had a busy day. I ask them to recognize that right now, in this moment, there is nowhere else they have to be, nothing else that needs to be done. They can give themselves permission to let go of planning, remembering, and figuring things out for the next few minutes.

Modeling the Mindfulness Process During the Exercise

As you listen to experienced MBCT and MBSR instructors lead exercises (e.g., Kabat-Zinn, 2012; Teasdale, Williams, & Segal, 2014; Woods, 2010), you will notice that they are not simply reading a list of directions. They are modeling the mindfulness process itself with their tone and their words. As clients listen, they will begin to internalize the attitude of openness, curiosity, exploration, and acceptance that develops through mindfulness practice.

With experience, you will develop your own personal style, but word choice can be very important. As an example, you might use a phrase like, "Noticing when your mind wanders, gently bringing it back, as best you can." "Noticing" is about breaking out of automatic pilot and models awareness. "When your mind wanders" normalizes getting lost in thoughts, modeling nonjudgment. "Gently bringing it back" models the attitude of kindness that is important to have with the discipline of reining in the attention. "As best you can" models the attitude of just doing what you can in each moment and not getting caught up in struggles, judgments, and comparisons.

You are actually doing the exercises yourself as you lead the group, but it is important to maintain several "meta-layers" of awareness, remembering where you are in the exercise and what the next instruction will be, keeping in mind the session's theme to know which points to emphasize, monitoring the group members, and noting things that may be important to inquire about and process afterward. In early sessions, the exercises may be shorter, with more structure. Toward the end of the course, clients can more comfortably sit longer, with less need for filling in the silence with detailed instructions.

I keep my eyes slightly open throughout all the exercises to monitor how the participants are doing. Are they shifting or fidgeting around a lot, perhaps due to pain or anxiety? Are heads bobbing from drifting into sleep? I will watch to see if these things change, or I may ask them to practice allowing their experiences to be however they find them, or I may talk about staying with and exploring difficulties, or I may end the exercise a little earlier to process their experiences.

Transitioning Out of the Exercise

I have been to places where the meditations were designed to take you to a different state of consciousness, so it took a while for people to come back into "normal" reality, and they often looked a little dazed and confused. Mindfulness is about waking up to this moment, so there should not be a dramatic shift when the exercise is over. Yet, especially when working internally with thoughts and difficulties, it can be helpful to allow a little time to ease people back to the group. "Being aware of sitting here, for just a few more moments. Now, gradually bringing your attention back to the room. Whenever you are ready, allowing your eyes to open, and moving or stretching your body if you like."

Zindel Segal (2013) suggests explicitly saying something like, "Noticing the transition, as we end this exercise and bring our awareness back to the room." Watching "transitions" between practices and between moments allows us to carry more of this quality of awareness and being present into the moments that follow.

Mindful Inquiry

The mindful inquiry process is perhaps the most crucial ingredient for leading successful MBCT groups, yet it is one of the biggest challenges for new therapists to learn. The concepts of mindful inquiry are well described in the protocol manual (Segal, Williams, & Teasdale, 2013) and by instructors such as Rebecca Crane (2009) and Susan Woods (2013). In what follows, I will touch on a few important considerations, and the transcripts will give some concrete examples of how the inquiry process plays out.

Attitude

When I was younger, I tried to learn as much as possible and push onto others what I thought was best for them. Now I just try to manifest being more present in my own life, which ironically turns out to be much more helpful to others. Attitude is very important in teaching mindfulness—the words you say are mostly forgotten, but the presence, the feeling of warmth and acceptance, is what the clients learn to internalize.

Jon Kabat-Zinn (2013) lists seven aspects of the attitudinal foundation of mindfulness practice: nonjudging, patience, beginner's mind, trust, nonstriving, acceptance, and letting go. These and other qualities are expanded upon by Crane (2009) and the original MBCT developers (Segal, Williams, & Teasdale, 2013).

The good news (and perhaps the bad news) is that there is no concrete formula for manifesting these qualities in the group. In fact, the harder you try, the more artificial you will seem. The qualities are natural "side effects" of regular mindfulness practice.

While traditional process-/relationship-oriented psychotherapy groups are very efficacious for a variety of issues (Corey, 2012; Yalom & Leszcz, 2005), MBCT groups have a different focus. They are about teaching and experiencing mindfulness skills. One of the most difficult things for a new MBCT therapist is to let go of the need to analyze or "fix" a participant's challenges. In the context of an MBCT group, trying to "figure out" and "fix" problems subtly models an inability to first stay with the situation as it is or implies that negative thoughts and feelings must immediately be pushed away. While engaged in the process of trying to fix a problem, we may be avoiding the emotions and body sensations that are already present, reinforcing a cycle of avoidance. If you or the other group members get caught up in trying to fix things, you can simply model coming back to what is actually happening in the present moment. "I'm noticing that we are all trying to give Joe advice. I'm wondering if we're all feeling a little helpless right now. What thoughts and feelings are coming up for everyone?" Or you can simply ask participants to do a 3-minute breathing space and move on with the class material.

When difficulties do come up in session during the inquiry stage, help the participants understand that being with a difficulty is itself practicing mindfulness, not a means to some altered state of consciousness. Model this by asking them what they noticed as they were nodding off, fidgeting, or whatever the difficulty was. Clients are often concerned about doing the exercises "right," which they usually interpret as meaning they should be always focused and peaceful.

Of course, do not throw away your clinical skills, just watch out for automatic habits. Be mindful of when to use and not use them. It can certainly be important at times to give information. If a clinical crisis comes up, you may need to shift into crisis intervention mode, but I have never found that necessary in all the groups I have done. However, there have been a number of occasions when I needed to check in with someone after class and sometimes make referrals for individual therapy.

One of the points emphasized in the group is that everything begins with noticing. Compulsively trying to push away difficulties lends itself to getting caught up in automatic reactions. When we explore things as they are and separate the situation from our thoughts, emotions, and sensations related to it, we will be much better equipped to make a conscious choice in how to proceed.

As an MBCT instructor, be careful not to judge the participants' experiences as "right" and "wrong." The person who notices his thoughts wandered continuously is practicing mindfulness just as much as someone who says her mind was clear throughout the entire exercise. Someone who noticed that he became relaxed is not "better" than the person who noticed her lower back was hurting. By getting more in touch with the moment as it is, we open up more possibilities for conscious responding. Mindfulness is not a "thing" that gives commands—it is a tool to foster awareness. Through practice, each person decides how to use it, what it means to them, and how they want to live their lives. We share suggestions that might be helpful, but basically our task is to shed light on the question, "How's that working for you?"

Three Layers of Inquiry

It can be useful to classify inquiry into three layers: noticing, exploring through discussion, and linking to daily life (Crane, 2009; Segal, Williams, & Teasdale, 2013; Woods, 2013). These three layers are embedded in the three questions that are asked upon completing a newly introduced mindfulness exercise.

The first question is, "What did you notice?" Asking this question, along with follow-up questions, provides participants a model for being dynamically mindful of their own experiences. This stage emphasizes awareness of direct experiences, disentangled from interpretations about them. Instructors model description versus judgment.

A very powerful piece of this stage is demonstrating the process of "decoupling" our experiences from our thoughts and feelings about them (Kabat-Zinn & Moyers, 1993; Kuyken et al., 2010). Participants discover that even though thoughts, emotions, and body sensations powerfully affect each other, they can be "uncoupled" from each other, or teased apart. This then gives us three places from which to work with something difficult.

From the very first session, we discuss the two ways of knowing—thinking and feeling (Segal & Lau, 2013; Segal, Williams, & Teasdale, 2013). Thinking about your feet is different than the experience of feeling your feet. The experience of mindfully eating a raisin is often very different from the thoughts we have about it. If someone says, "I remembered how much I hate raisins!" the instructor can observe, "So, you noticed a thought came up that you hate raisins. Was there an emotion or body sensation present? Were you able to bring your attention back to the raisin? What did you notice about the raisin? Did you decide to eat it, or not eat it?"

It can also be helpful to invite discussion from others, particularly if participants don't speak up right away or if one person tends to dominate the discussions. "Did anyone else notice something similar to what Jane described?" "Many of you said you feel more relaxed now. Did anyone have the opposite experience, maybe feeling more upset than you did before you stopped to notice?"

The second question is, "How is what we just did different from the way you might normally . . . (eat, relate to your body, walk, etc.)?" This question helps foster awareness of automatic patterns and how bringing more mindfulness into daily experiences affects those patterns.

The third question is, "What do you think this exercise has to do with why you are here (depression, stress, pain, etc.)?" This is the question everyone is thinking, so it is important to make it explicit. The average client will not go on faith that if they practice for years, it will all come to them. It is crucial to tie the exercise to something very practical for their daily lives.

Whenever possible, let the process itself teach the participants, or let the participants learn from hearing about each other's experiences. Resist the urge to fall into a continual mode of telling them everything. Neophyte instructors can get so excited about their new discoveries that they want to tell everyone. It is certainly okay to share insights, but it has a deeper impact when they experience it. Rather than telling them in words, set up the exercises and inquiry process to help them experience it. Watch out for setting yourself up to be an expert on everything, where everyone looks to you for the "final word" or the "right" way to do it. This kills curiosity, which is what we want to foster. I am often amazed at the brilliant insights that participants bring up if I allow them the time and space. When they are paying attention, they are the experts when it comes to their own experiences.

Of course, don't avoid direct questions either, implying that they have to work hard to get the "secret." You can always bring up important points when asked or if no one else does. If people all seem to be going off in an unhelpful direction, such as thinking that ignoring pain by focusing on the breath is the only option for dealing with it, then it is important to make some suggestions, like, "I wonder what would happen if you . . ." or "next time you might explore . . ."

The inquiry process should ideally be modified to highlight the themes of the particular session (Segal & Lau, 2013). For example, if someone mentions they were in pain during an exercise in the first session (Awareness and Automatic Pilot), you might highlight noticing and teasing apart thoughts, emotions, and sensations. In session five (Allowing/Letting Be), you might highlight experimenting with staying present with the experience, which they might normally push away immediately.

Use of Stories and Humor

Mindfulness concepts can be challenging to convey through analytical explanation. This is why there is such an emphasis on practice and inquiry. In addition, the protocol suggests the use of poems, analogies, and stories to communicate some of the important principles (Segal, Williams, & Teasdale, 2013).

In my experience, if I go on with lengthy explanations, the words begin to lose their meaning, and the eyes of the participants begin to glaze over. However, stories can convey more subtleties and are more likely to engage participants. Initially, I mostly used examples and stories from the manual, other books, and other instructors. Gradually, I could speak more directly from my own experiences and was able to tailor examples to the particular experiences and issues of the participants in the group.

Humor can also be important if used appropriately. The often serious topics of discussion can be delivered with a lightness of touch. Be mindful of occasions when humor is overused, perhaps to avoid something difficult or when it becomes offensive. A quick scan of the participants' faces will let you know how your humor is being perceived.

Humor toward oneself can be especially helpful, as it models acceptance. Once, I went to take a quick drink of water as I was giving a talk on mindfulness in front of 200 mental health professionals, squeezed my water bottle too hard, and completely soaked the front of my shirt. There was no hiding it, and nothing to be done. I smiled and said, "Okay, I'm going to feel the embarrassment, allow it rise up, level off, and pass away." Everyone laughed, and we could then move on without trying to pretend it never happened.

Self-Disclosure

MBCT leaders are also participants in the group, so sharing what you notice during an exercise models an open sense of curiosity and exploration. It also helps others feel comfortable doing this for themselves and gives them examples of how to do it. This is most helpful in the earlier stages of the group. Eventually, most groups do so well with this that instructors share less and less so as not to take away time from the participants.

As in other professional situations, always ask yourself if what you are sharing will be helpful to the group rather than just using the group as therapy for yourself. If you share too much about a struggle you are having, the group may turn the focus on you. On the other hand, sharing your own challenges shows the group that no one is perfect at doing this practice and can serve as a model for allowing yourself to feel and experience difficulties without them overwhelming you.

Keep a balance between keeping hope that this practice is helpful and showing that you don't have to be perfect. If you brag too much about how hard mindfulness is for you, the clients will become discouraged. I tend to share a little more of my human failings toward the end of the course, when the clients have already had their own experiences and can relate better to the challenges and how helpful the mindfulness practices can be.

As instructors, we may sometimes feel like frauds. After all, we know darn well that our lives are not perfect, that we still have ups and downs, that we occasionally still get hooked by thoughts. But we also want to provide inspiration. So, as a brand new MBCT leader, you might not say out loud, "Wow, I am feeling really terrified that I'm not doing this right!" It may be better to model just staying present, pausing, and responding carefully. Of course, for very challenging questions, it is also fine to simply say, "I don't know, that's a good question," or "I'm not sure, let me do some research on that," then rein the group back in to the curriculum.

Working With Challenging Participants

In most of my groups, everyone is there with an open mind, seeking personal growth or relief from their symptoms. However, when you are a new group leader, it is common to fear the worst scenarios and to be concerned about how you might handle them.

Since one of the primary goals of these groups is to notice reality as it is, it is usually not good to ignore challenging clients. It may sound like a paradox to model acceptance and nonjudgment while actively keeping the group on track, but acceptance does not mean whatever happens is fine. You can model acceptance and still be proactive, even setting firm boundaries about appropriate behavior in the group when necessary.

It is especially important to recognize how our biases can contribute to perceptions of what makes for a "difficult" client. It can be helpful to remember that the root problems for these clients come from difficult thoughts, feelings, and sensations. Many times, challenges come from fear, from lack of understanding, or from not feeling understood. Just being present with their thoughts and feelings is very powerful. Avoid giving them platitudes or implying that there is something wrong with them for having the thoughts and feelings they have or presenting mindfulness as if it is some kind of cornucopia of bliss and happiness.

While "challenging" clients intimidate new therapists, eventually you may come to really enjoy working with them. After all, it is an indication that the clients are feeling safe, accepted, engaged, and working to make the material personally meaningful for themselves. The bottom line is that you keep doing the same thing. You do not treat challenging clients differently. Be sure that you are present with each participant as best you can be. Be careful of talking about acceptance but subtly sneering, rolling your eyes, or avoiding certain clients. Make sure that you are not giving the appearance of aligning with the other members and attacking or rejecting the challenging client.

Make the environment safe and comfortable for asking challenging questions. Avoid getting defensive in your answers, perhaps saying, "I don't know the answer to your question, but I can find out," or "In my experience, you will come to discover what works best for you after you experiment a little." Model the mindful attitude of acceptance and nonjudgment that you are teaching. This modeling can be far more powerful than any words you use. Thank them for such questions.

Here is where your own personal practice will become crucial. Just as our thoughts can grab us and tell us they are true with strong conviction, so too will participants hook us. Though it can present a challenge for new facilitators, it provides a crucial opportunity for participants to learn a new way to stay present with difficult thoughts and emotions. We can deal with difficult clients the same way we have learned to deal with our own difficult feelings, sensations, and thoughts through our own personal practice. We can become like catalysts, sparking reactions with our presence but not being used up in the process.

We learn from the participants. We are not above them. We are sharing a journey. Participants often come up with amazing stories, fascinating insights, and even very challenging questions that can actually lead to significant growth for the therapist as well as the other participants.

Even though you are a fellow human being on the path and should not act is if you are superior to the participants, in this setting, your role is to be the leader. You may sometimes need to be very active to address concerns, to interrupt inappropriate intrusions into a group member's personal business, or to actively bring the group back to task when it goes too far astray. How you handle difficult situations in the here and now of the group may be far more valuable than anything you can say with words.

Just as we do in our practice, we can notice when things go off topic and bring the participants gently back to task. Digressions, just like mind wandering, can sometimes be a way of avoiding a challenging or uncomfortable experience. Most of us were raised to believe that polite people do not interrupt, but we can do this skillfully. "I'm noticing that we keep drifting off the subject. Let's do a 3-minute breathing space and come back to this moment." When working with children using MBCT-C, we can just ring the "bells of mindfulness" (Semple & Lee, 2011).

Remember also the concept of shifting between process and content (Corey, 2012; Yalom & Leszcz, 2005). New clinicians often automatically get caught up in the content of the questions or problem. Shifting to a process, such as noticing that the question actually stems from a need to control one's feelings, can be helpful to make the discussion more productive. Of course, this must be done in a balanced way, or clients will feel like you are being shifty and avoiding answering their questions.

Though I have never had to do this, it is conceivable that you may need to ask a member to leave if they are not benefitting and are undermining the rest of the group or that they might benefit more from the group after doing some individual work. However, before this point, you may have a golden opportunity to open up new ways of being for the challenging member and model healthier ways of dealing with difficult relationships for the other group members.

While of course important for all aspects of clinical practice, awareness and training in cultural and other diversity issues is especially crucial in working with someone who seems like a "difficult" client. For example, "silent clients" may simply be showing deference to authority and may be uncomfortable expressing too much about themselves.

In practice, you will seldom see individuals exactly like those described in what follows, as all behaviors lie on a continuum. Most groups do not have any "problem" clients, and the most I've had in any one group has been two or three, and the groups were still very successful. That said, when supervising new MBCT therapists, questions often come up about how to work with clients like those described below.

Health Care Professionals

Many of my groups have a large percentage of health professionals in them for their own personal growth or stress reduction or because they are hoping to learn something they can use with patients. Many of them may have an automatic tendency to want to help others, give them advice, or question the evidence base. Though I may address these things, I find that they usually fade after the first couple of sessions, after they become more comfortable with letting go of those automatic reactions and practicing for themselves.

I personally greatly enjoy having health professionals in the group. For new MBCT therapists, the biggest "problem" may be self-doubt. Just remember you do not have to be "better" than the other therapists or physicians in the group. You are simply offering a place to share skills and experiences.

Business Professionals

If you have not worked in the fast-paced world of business, you might be intimidated by the directness and need for practicality of many executives. Below is a short and direct email I received from a CEO halfway through an MBCT course, followed by my response:

> *"I am having trouble (time) doing the homework. What else can I work on to make this course worth my time?"*
>
> In the big picture of things, you have to make a decision that you are worth it. I've already seen how non-stop your mind is working, which is helpful for your business, but will likely take a long-term toll on your health. Even from a practical perspective, having more clarity of mind will help you work more efficiently in the future.
>
> I would suggest at least trying the 3-minute breathing space track, before you go to sleep, and at other times of the day if you can.
>
> I also find it best to 'make an appointment' for the practice, ideally the same time each day, so you don't have to decide when to do it, and so that it doesn't get forgotten.
>
> You can even make the not doing it part of the practice—try to notice what you are thinking and feeling when you make the decision not to do it.
>
> This can be a very difficult new habit to start, but eventually works its way naturally into your life.

The "bottom line" question that I find helpful for most business professionals is, "Is what you are doing right now sustainable?" As we have learned from motivational interviewing (Miller & Rollnick, 2013), trying to talk someone into something only builds resistance, and it models lack of acceptance. If someone wants to quit, you can tell them that they certainly could choose to do so if they feel they are wasting their time, but it seems that this very feeling of being forever rushed and never finished, always lost in thoughts about what needs to be done or what happened, has been creating serious problems for them, and moving into and investigating these patterns opens more possibility for creating a shift.

The Advice Giver/Cotherapist

Interpersonal learning and feedback are very powerful in traditional process-oriented group therapy, allowing clients to feel helpful to others, to feel supported, and to get honest feedback (Corey, 2012; Yalom & Leszcz, 2005). However, this is deemphasized in MBCT. In this context, advice giving subtly models that we do not accept reality as it is, and it must be "fixed." It can also be a subtle way of avoiding present-moment experiences. While the facilitator need not squelch this every time, it is more useful to shift away from the content of the advice and notice the process. "It sounds like you feel a connection with Joe for what he is going through and want to offer something to help. Are you feeling some sadness yourself right now? Are others in the group remembering a difficult time and feeling it right now in your body?" How you proceed depends on the theme for that particular group. You could tie it into how thoughts affect feelings, the difficulty of accepting our experiences, or pause with a 3-minute breathing space and move on.

The Experienced Meditator

Most often, it is a delight to have experienced meditation practitioners, as they are usually open to learning from each moment. However, some may feel a need to prove themselves to others or to project a sense that their presence is a blessing to the others in the group and that they don't really need the class themselves. Model acceptance and nonjudgment for these individuals as best you can, bringing it back to the moment. "So you were noticing yourself thinking about your previous experiences. What were you aware of in your body during this exercise?"

There are many forms of meditation, so it is important to recognize the differences. It is not about mindfulness being "better" than other forms but about being conscious of what you are doing. On occasion, someone with a background in an absorption type of meditation will say they "went off" into a blissful, altered state of consciousness. I will ask them, "Did you do that on purpose?" It is also a useful skill to choose to remain present when things are difficult. It would not be helpful to "go off" into altered consciousness if you are having an argument with your partner.

As an MBCT instructor, learning about and practicing other forms of meditation can broaden your understanding of them and can help you relate to the broad and varied practices participants will bring up as they compare what they have done in the past to the practice of mindfulness. As a word of caution, some meditation practices are best learned under the guidance of a competent instructor. As with mindfulness, we can inadvertently end up spending a lot of time mistakenly practicing something that is very different than what the meditation is designed for.

It is even possible to run into some serious difficulties. Once in a while, clients come to me for individual therapy to help them understand frightening experiences they have had from certain practices. How a person reacts to these bizarre mental experiences can make them worse. Having a competent teacher helps to prepare for and process these experiences in a productive way. Sometimes clients have these experiences due to the influence of substances or may be developing or suffering from a thought disorder.

"Eccentric" Clients

Sometimes participants may seem a bit "odd," perhaps in the way they interact with others, the spiritual ideas they present, or in holding on to beliefs that some would consider strange. Since the group is not about adopting a set of beliefs, there is no need to get into debates. Individuals may come into the groups with mild thought disorders, neurocognitive disorders, or autism spectrum disorders. As always, model noticing, acceptance, and patience, bringing the group back to task rather than engaging in philosophical debates.

The Naysayer

This is the person most feared by new therapists, the one who openly challenges you, the one with strong opinions. Perhaps they shoot things down, saying that it just won't work for them, a client Yalom calls the "help-rejecting complainer" (Yalom & Leszcz, 2005).

Consider the exchange I had with a veteran with PTSD halfway through our MBCT sessions:

"So what did you notice during that exercise?"

"I just kept thinking this is bullshit! How is this supposed to be helping me?"

"So you noticed lots of thoughts about this being bullshit. Were you able to notice what your body was feeling once in a while?"

"Sometimes. But I just couldn't stop thinking about how this was bullshit, and whether or not I should be honest with you about that."

"So you noticed that while you were thinking, you were only vaguely aware of what you were actually experiencing."

As I modeled simply noticing what was happening instead of getting defensive, the client went on exploring his own experiences. After a few minutes, he said that in fact, he was able to enjoy being present with his grandchildren more and noticed that he didn't worry as much as he used to, so maybe this stuff was helping him.

I have had clients say that it is simply not possible to make time for practicing or begin to get cynical about mindfulness itself. I never get into arguments about whether or not to "believe" in mindfulness. I come back to the point that everything starts with noticing. Mindfulness doesn't tell you what to do, it just helps you make more informed decisions about what to do. One of the most helpful questions is, "How have things been working for you up to this point?" or some variation.

Chances are, the cynical person does not have very good relationships. Chances are, the people who are too busy to practice are feeling very overwhelmed and are setting themselves up for a crash. Will they be satisfied with those results?

Of course you must set appropriate boundaries, especially if a group member is making others uncomfortable, but modeling awareness and acceptance of all present-moment experiences, even "negative" ones, is very powerful for all of the participants. Very often, the naysayers are the ones who thank me the most at the end of the 8 weeks.

The Groupie

Lying at the other end of the continuum is the "groupie," who hangs on your every word, laughs a little too loudly at all your jokes, and wants to impress you. This person may believe that mindfulness is the panacea for all the world's ills and revere mindfulness as if it had a capital "M."

In addition to modeling acceptance, invite these clients to investigate their own experiences, asking them about their body sensations, emotions, and/or thoughts. I also find humor helpful. After several occasions of a particular woman laughing much too loudly at my jokes, I began saying, "buh-dum-pah!" as if giving myself a drum fill.

Though it can be challenging, we are continually balancing the concrete, practical, and realistic aspects of mindfulness with the hope and inspiration that clients need to practice a new approach to relating to their lives.

The Silent Client

In interpersonal process group psychotherapy, silent clients tend not to benefit from the group and can eventually damage group cohesion (Yalom & Leszcz, 2005). However, given the class-based focus of MBCT, participants are informed that they do not have to speak, although they are more likely to benefit from active participation.

When a normally silent client does speak up, be sure to acknowledge it, even if only with body language. Have you ever said something difficult to a group of people, and no one even seemed to notice? It may have made you regret you said anything at all. On the other hand, some clients may want to share but feel like what they have to say is not important enough, and they may respond well to encouragement.

I tend not to call on particular individuals, though I may look at someone and raise my eyebrows in invitation if they look as though they have something to say. Be careful not to put someone on the spot with too many follow-up questions, or they may be afraid to speak up again. It is best to ask permission to probe further (Segal, Williams, & Teasdale, 2013). "May I ask you a little more about that? Where did you feel that in your body? Did you notice any changes over the course of the exercise?"

Stuck in the Past/Acutely Depressed

Some clients may frequently bring up past events. As therapists, it can be easy to get caught up in delving deeper into the past, but in MBCT groups, this tends to be counterproductive. There is no end to analyzing past events. Instead, we can bring things back to the present moment, as we hope the client will begin to do more often, by asking, "As you were describing that event, were you aware of any feelings coming up now, in this moment? Are you noticing any familiar thought patterns?"

As we know, ruminations about the past are characteristic of acute depression. Individuals in the group with acute or residual depression may end up "falling behind" the others as the weeks go on (Segal, 2008). When you are depressed, it is difficult to muster the cognitive capacity to do the work of practicing mindfulness. Frank discussions with the client after class may be necessary to determine if the person should continue or if it would be better to seek individual therapy before coming back for a future group.

Stuck in the Future/Anxious

Patrick McGrath (2013) defines anxiety as "What if," followed by all the worst possible things that could happen. He observes that no one ever worries about, "What if everything goes my way today?" It is natural to struggle with worry, as the brain has a tendency to look for what could go wrong. If we can anticipate and prepare for future danger, we can survive longer to reproduce. Our brains can come up with fantastic possibilities for how disaster could strike, even if very improbable. Trying to talk ourselves out of the resulting anxiety is often what keeps us stuck. We may even have very real reasons to be worried about the future, such as an upcoming medical test or court date, and we may tell ourselves that we "must" worry.

Remember that all this thinking is our brain's way of trying to help, by distracting us from our anxiety in the moment. We don't quite feel it as much when we are off in our heads. Clients who report feeling "antsy," who are shifting around in their chairs, are also often doing so to fight their habit of "doing something" to avoid the feelings of anxiety. As with exposure therapy, sitting with our experiences rather than avoiding them allows them to rise and fall on their own.

Another form of being stuck in the future is as an attempt to escape dealing with unpleasant current situations. Holding on to the idea that things are all going to be great "someday" is another way of getting temporary relief from current emotions like grief and depression.

Facilitators should watch out for getting hooked by these traps and model the mindfulness process in the present moment of the session. "So you're noticing that you are thinking a lot. What are you feeling in your body right now?" Chances are, there will be some underlying sensations related to anxiety. The group offers a safe space for clients to move into their experiences in a more direct way, separating their thoughts from their emotions and body sensations. Realizing that moving directly into unpleasant body sensations can change and even extinguish them, even if there is first an "extinction burst," is a very powerful insight.

Addictions

Addictions are something we all have to varying degrees, whether to coffee, TV shows, or certain routines. While mindfulness-based relapse prevention focuses specifically on treating addictive behaviors (Bowen, Chawla, &

Marlatt, 2010), substance use and other addictive disorders are often comorbid with individuals struggling with stress, anxiety, and depression. It is therefore important to be comfortable working with addiction-related issues.

While addictions are very challenging, a general principle to keep in mind is that the addictive behavior is mainly used to manage feelings. Taking a substance or engaging in a particular behavior serves to take away something unpleasant, such as cravings or stress. When cravings or thoughts of using come up, one can learn to sit with them, allowing them to rise and fall on their own. Mindfulness is not about taking away the urges but helps clients learn to move into them, relate to them differently, and ride them out (Bowen, Chawla, & Marlatt, 2010).

Traumas

Mindfulness work with individuals who have PTSD must be done very carefully and requires special expertise (Sears & Chard, 2015). However, given the high percentage of individuals who have experienced trauma, it is inevitable that these issues will come up, even if they are not identified as the primary presenting issues.

Very strong emotions may come up for some individuals. Recently, after doing the body scan in a first session and asking the class, "What did you notice?" one woman said, "I felt my foot, but hearing your voice and feeling my body was freaking me out. I had an urge to run out of the room. I just zoned out for most of it." I immediately suspected trauma, so I chose not to ask for details, simply observing, "So you were aware of strong feelings and a desire to run out of the room, but you chose to stay."

Interestingly, a member of the same group asked me questions after class about the concept of choosing to shift to awareness of feelings when strong thoughts are present. "But I can't feel anything," she said. And yet, I observed out loud that as she was speaking to me, her eyes were tearing up, so she was obviously feeling something. Perhaps she had taught herself not to notice her feelings as a way of making it through tough times.

It is important to proceed carefully when trauma issues come up. Education about the general nature of trauma can be helpful to the group, but it is not appropriate to delve into the details of personal history in the context of an MBCT group, and the leader should proactively shift from content to process when this starts to happen. Referral may be necessary. In both of the examples just mentioned, the individuals confirmed with me that they were already working with individual therapists and were looking to add mindfulness as a tool for their work.

Training and Supervising Students

Because there is currently a dearth of qualified MBCT instructors, you may soon find yourself supervising others who wish to learn. Taking on students is a big responsibility that should not be taken lightly. In addition to having skills and experience with MBCT, it is important to have training in providing clinical supervision. I commonly hear complaints from students that their supervisors are good clinicians but lousy supervisors, and I often see state boards giving sanctions for problems related to supervision. There are many good books and workshops on this topic (e.g., Bernard & Goodyear, 2014; Falender & Shafranske, 2004).

I found that my own growth and competence increased exponentially after taking on students, and they keep me learning. Having students present brings more conscious awareness to how I run the groups and helps me to clarify ways of expressing concepts. Students also provide fresh perspectives, fascinating insights, and up-to-date research findings.

It is helpful to meet with the students a few minutes after each session to process how the group went. Far from being a "secret" meeting, I let the participants know about this and let them know they are welcome to stay if they like. As Yalom (2006) notes, the meta-processing that occurs with students while clients are present can be very helpful.

Of course, the supervisor can model present-moment, nonjudgmental acceptance of student thoughts, questions, and concerns. Ask them what they noticed about particular participants. Was anyone not engaged or struggling? Do the clients seem to be getting the principles? Which clients might be pulling or "hooking" me or the student? I also share, in an appropriate way, any thoughts or feelings that come up for me, any times I noticed myself getting hooked, and the choices I made. As with the group itself, this modeling is far more valuable than any clever intellectual insights I could try to invent.

Have the students go through the group just like all the other participants, doing homework and participating. Don't let them sit "outside" the group as "observers." As with group members, it becomes noticeable which students are practicing on their own and when they are starting to embody rather than imitate the principles. Gradually have the student become more active in the group. Start off with having them lead mindfulness practices and topic discussions, then practicing inquiry. When a student is leading, resist the urge to take over unless something important needs to be clarified. Once students lead groups on their own, it can be helpful to get client permission to record the sessions to give students feedback.

Practicalities

Once you are ready to begin offering MBCT groups, there are a number of important practicalities to consider before getting started.

Setting

Ideally, you want to foster a setting and atmosphere conducive to facilitating mindfulness skills. In many cases, you may simply be assigned a room in an agency or a hospital and will have to make do with whatever you are given.

To begin with, carefully consider the cultural and spiritual backgrounds of the clients in your region. It may be best to display natural, inspiring objects or images rather than decorations that suggest a particular spirituality. Soft lighting is preferable to overly bright, harsh industrial lights, though there needs to be enough light for everyone to remain awake and to easily read the handouts.

Ideally, the setting should be fairly quiet, with a comfortable temperature, and free of distractions. However, since distractions are inevitable in most places, these can be used as opportunities for noticing how our minds react to them.

I find it best to provide chairs for everyone, with cushions available for those who prefer to sit on the floor. Otherwise, clients may think they should imitate the teacher by sitting on the floor and may end up with sore backs and sore legs, impeding their attention.

Preparing for the Group

A little preparation is necessary before each group, though ideally this can be taken care of early on. Wonderfully, the protocol manual contains all the handouts for the entire course (Segal, Williams, & Teasdale, 2013). When printing them, you may wish to add a customized cover page listing such things as the facility name and your name and contact information. While the audios are now available as free downloads as well, I make a number of audio CDs to give those with less computer savvy.

Some sessions require specific items, such as raisins, stones, or marker boards. The original protocol required audio/visual equipment to show a video, though this is no longer necessary.

Most importantly, allow enough time for your own personal preparation for the session. Allow yourself plenty of time to arrange the space, organize your materials, and ground yourself in the present moment.

Time Management

Most MBCT instructors allow between 2 and 3 hours for each session. I have found this to be taxing for the working individuals in my evening groups, so I cover the material in 90 minutes. While I have always received positive feedback, I am conducting more controlled research on how effective shorter sessions are. My guided meditations are shortened to 20 to 30 minutes, and there are times when the inquiry process is not as long as I would like it to be.

Initially, it may be helpful to keep the agenda for the session next to you, with notes on what time each segment should begin and end, to stay on track with time. With experience, you will get a feel for each segment of each session. While flexibility to adapt to the current group and their needs is important, you should mindfully choose if you want to stay with any given segment longer rather than being surprised when people begin walking out of the room when it is time to end.

Marketing

It can be a challenge generating momentum to gather enough interest to start MBCT groups. For the first few years, I held groups in my private practice, and it was considerable work to find enough people. For the past several years, I have had great success in partnering with integrative health agencies. The agency provides the space, marketing, and referrals, collects the fees, and writes me a check after taking percentage.

Marketing options expand when you plan ahead with dates for the groups, ideally at regular, predictable times. You may need to experiment with the hours and days that work best for you and the population you wish to serve.

Remember that the best marketing is often free. Local publications and media are often grateful for articles and interviews about stress and mental health. There are often opportunities to give presentations to schools and organizations, which can lead to interest in the groups and sometimes even contracts to provide groups at their locations.

Letters, flyers, and/or direct contacts with other health care providers can be very helpful. I sometimes allow health professionals to attend the groups for free so they feel more comfortable sending referrals. Offering continuing-education credits is also an incentive for health providers to attend.

A professionally designed and regularly maintained website is also very important to provide information and credibility. My own website, www.psych-insights.com, contains a video of a brief talk I gave about mindfulness. Clients have often told me that they enjoyed the video, shared it with friends, and became intrigued to learn more. Some may still find it strange to commit to an 8-week meditation program, so seeing a face and making a connection with a person, even if only through video, can be very helpful. It also establishes you as a competent authority and dispels any potential worries about getting into something odd or cultish.

Reimbursement

There are a number of possible reimbursement options, depending upon your region and the population with whom you are working. For the general groups that I do for the public, I have had the most success in collecting the entire fee before or on the first day of the course. Collecting a fee for each session can become a hassle, create awkward moments, or even contribute to someone quitting. Once they have joined the group, I explicitly joke with clients that we ask for their money up front so they will not quit when it gets challenging.

I have also found it helpful to give a discount for those who register in advance. For those with significant financial challenges, I offer a "scholarship," allowing them to come for half price or even pro bono. I also frequently allow graduate students to attend at no charge. I enjoy working with them, and if they have attended several and "get it," they can cover a session for me in case of illness.

Some third-party payers may reimburse as group psychotherapy if a diagnosis is provided. Frankly, I prefer to avoid the hassle of all the ramifications this entails since I promote the groups as skill-building, psychoeducational sessions.

Recordkeeping

Documentation considerations will depend on the relevant local laws for your profession, the setting, and the population. In any case, it is important to provide each participant with informed consent.

If I am using the MBCT protocol with an individual, I clarify up front if they are looking for "private lessons" for the mindfulness skills only or seeing this as a part of individual psychotherapy. In my experience, people often come privately because they are dealing with major life issues, so I document the sessions as psychotherapy.

If you are conducting the groups in a medical setting or are billing third-party payers for the sessions as group psychotherapy for a mental health diagnosis such as major depressive disorder, good practice recommends keeping separate notes on each individual, with a general summary of how each group session went (APA, 2007). If you conduct the group as an educational class, you may not be required to keep detailed records.

Ongoing Groups

As is explicitly discussed in session eight, without ongoing practice, one can slip back into old patterns of living on automatic pilot. Participants often express a desire to continue meeting, which can be helpful to inspire regular practice.

There are a variety of options, depending on the availability of the facilitator and the interest of the participants. Ideally, one can schedule regular "drop-in groups," where program graduates can come to do a mindfulness exercise together and discuss how their practices are going. One could also offer a "mindful lunch" session, eating in silence and doing a short exercise together before returning to work. Both the MBSR and MBCT protocol (Kabat-Zinn, 2013; Segal, Williams, & Teasdale, 2013) recommend holding a day of mindful practice between sessions six and seven, to which one invites past graduates. I have had a number of participants repeat the entire course, reporting that they got a lot more out of the class the second time through it. There may also be friendly local meditation groups that hold regular silent meditation practice sessions. Ongoing groups can even meet "virtually" through online video rooms.

Now that we have covered a variety of important MBCT concepts and techniques, let's look at the transcripts of an actual group for examples of how they might play out in each session.

Part II
Session Transcripts

4 The Initial Session

As with other types of group work, an initial meeting before the group begins serves a number of important purposes (Segal, Williams, & Teasdale, 2013; Yalom & Leszcz, 2005). It allows potential participants a chance to get to know the instructor, provides a big-picture overview of what the course is all about, and clarifies the expectations and commitment needed for home practice between the sessions. Like the social psychology phenomenon of a group seeming more attractive when it is difficult to get into, I find that letting them know they should probably not attend unless they can make a commitment to themselves to do the home practice and complete all eight sessions has the effect of a paradoxical strategic intervention.

Ideally, the initial session is conducted as an individual interview. This is detailed in the MBCT manual (Segal, Williams, & Teasdale, 2013). For this particular group, I chose to do the initial session in the form of a didactic presentation. There are pros and cons to this approach. Marketing a free stress-reduction workshop can be useful to attract potential participants and is much more time effective than meeting with each person individually. However, one cannot build meaningful rapport as well, and one does not gather as much background information on the client as one would from an individual interview.

Of note, I tend not to use MBCT in the title for a group like the one transcribed here, though I tell anyone who asks that I use that protocol. These groups are not like typical interpersonal "therapy" groups, as they are conducted more like educational, experiential, skill-building groups. I advertise the group mainly as a way of dealing with stress, since that is a common factor in many different presenting issues, emphasizing that mindfulness is a way of wisely working with our thoughts, emotions, and body sensations.

The reader will notice an emphasis here on working with stress, anxiety, depression, and other problems. While mindfulness is definitely also a tool for enriching your life, in my professional experience, people are not ready to hear that when they are suffering a lot. It will sound as if I am giving them pie-in-the-sky platitudes and not being realistic or not understanding where they are coming from. For wonderful examples of presenting mindfulness to the public with a balanced attitude that is concrete and practical yet moving and inspiring, I highly recommend the work of Jon Kabat-Zinn (e.g., 1994, 2006, 2013).

As with the group sessions themselves, the transcript that follows is not necessarily the best way to do an initial session and certainly is not meant to be memorized. It is meant to serve as one particular example, allowing you to catch of glimpse of what it would be like. Though I cover the same basic content each time, using computer-projected presentation slides, every initial session is adapted to fit the particular questions and needs of the audience. Before making a commitment, the attendees in my community often want to know details about the course, how it is different from other approaches, and why it works. They also want to make sure the facilitator is competent and personable.

Near the beginning of this talk, I gave an opportunity for people to express something about what they were looking for, but no one took it. Since this is a free public talk, people may not feel comfortable expressing anything personal, so I'm careful not to pressure anyone to speak. Likewise, after guiding the audience through the 3-minute breathing space, no one offered to describe their experience. In a class, I would have taken more time, asked it another way, or described my own experience to get the discussion rolling. However, since this was a free information session, and I could pick up that several of these individuals had some anxiety, I decided not to push them to share.

Initial Information Session Transcript

Dr. Sears: Let me start off saying I much prefer these to be interactive, so feel free to ask questions or make comments as we go. I actually like being challenged. Instead of just going along with everything I say, I'd much prefer, "Why wouldn't we do it this way?" or "How would this fit for me?" or "My life is different, and I tried this and it didn't work." Because then it becomes alive and workable and usable in your life, instead of just going along or trying to imitate someone else. For stress reduction, you don't want to take on something that causes more stress than it helps, right? You don't want to add 20 things you gotta do every day to reduce your stress—that can create more stress! The whole point of this is to bring it into your life in a natural way. We'll be talking about changing the way you *relate* to circumstances.

I should also say that this intro session is different from how we run the group itself. I'll be throwing a lot of information at you today. Since I mostly teach for a living, I'll drop more into professor mode, giving facts and data and background. I find that for a lot people, before committing to something, it helps to know a little about how and why mindfulness works. But the groups are going to be a lot more experiential, in terms of practicing the mindfulness exercises together, processing our experiences, and discussing how we can apply it in our daily lives. We'll do a brief exercise later to give you a taste of it.

I'm jumping ahead of myself already, but this is not a therapy group in the sense of talking about past hurts or telling secrets. It's more of a skill-building group for how you can apply this stuff in your life. For example, someone may share, "I noticed I was at work, and the boss said 'I need to see you in my office,' and suddenly I got really anxious." We might then talk about what you noticed during that experience, discuss how the concepts and practices from the class helped or didn't help, and explore other ways of relating to the experience. So the sharing is more about using the skills rather than revealing personal information. In fact, you could choose to go through the whole group and never say a word. You probably won't get very much out of it if you never talk, but you certainly won't be forced to participate.

Maybe I should back up and introduce myself. My name is Richard Sears, and I'm a psychologist by profession. I'm a professor in a doctoral program, where I teach other people how to become psychologists. I also have a small private practice where I'm actively working with clients, and I do mindfulness groups here. My way into this work is kind of funny, because it began when I was a teenager and got involved in the martial arts. I was lucky enough to have teachers who emphasized self-development, and the importance of the mind, instead of focusing on hurting people. I became interested in meditation and Eastern traditions, and delved deeply into that. When I opened a martial arts school and offered meditation classes, a few people began paying me for private lessons, but spent most of the time telling me their life problems, like how depressed they felt, or how bad their relationships were. I listened, but I wasn't very well equipped to deal with those issues. That drove me to become a psychologist and to get the science of how the mind works. As I immersed myself in psychology and cutting-edge brain science, I was fascinated to find so many similarities to what I'd been learning in the meditative traditions, just spoken in a different language. It was good timing for me career-wise, because the research on mindfulness has really been exploding. So that's me.

Are there any preliminary questions, or does anyone want to throw something out about what they're looking for?

Laura: I have a little bit of a hearing problem, so if you could speak just a little bit louder that would be great.

Dr. Sears: Okay, sure, just raise a finger if I get too quiet. Anything else before we jump into this stuff?

First of all, I want to talk a little bit about stress. Even here on the flyer for this group we have a list of many of the things mindfulness has been shown to help. It starts to look like some kind of "snake oil" thing, as if this will cure all these different conditions. But we're really talking about stress as a common factor for all these problems, which creates a negative cascade effect on your body and your nervous system, contributing to or leaving you more vulnerable to mental and physical issues. It's not that mindfulness magically cures these specific problems necessarily, but by managing stress, and making more conscious choices, it can help with a wide variety of challenges.

Before we start talking about reducing stress, it's important to recognize that a little stress is actually a good thing. I don't know if any of you took statistics, or have seen Selye's curve before (Selye, 1976), but this curve here means if my stress is low, then my performance is actually low. Having some stress actually gives you energy and motivation to accomplish things. If you really had no stress, you might not even get out of bed or do anything, although I'm sure some of you are thinking that you'd like to see what it would be like to have no stress [laughter].

Most of us, though, can more easily identify with the other side, where high stress also leads to low performance. You're overwhelmed, you've got too much going on, you can't think straight, you're feeling this constant sense of rushing around, and you're working harder but you're not getting more done. Optimally, we want to find a balance here in the middle, where there's some stress in our lives, but it's not overwhelming.

When we talk about the stress response, it's important to think about how this is actually a good thing. In the short term, the stress response is designed to help us survive a momentary situation. If a lion suddenly appears at the door, unless you're some kind of cold-blooded lion killer, we will all have an immediate response, sparked by our sympathetic nervous system. Adrenaline and cortisol get released into your bloodstream. Your heart pumps harder and faster, so your blood pressure goes up to get

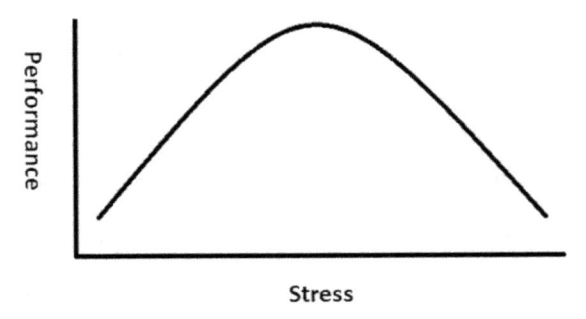

Figure 4.1 Stress curve

more oxygen to the muscles so we can run fast, hopefully at least faster than the person next to you [laughter]. If you're running for your life from a lion, not much need to digest your food or reproduce at that moment, so the blood flow to your digestive and reproductive organs decreases to give more to the muscles.

In fact, I once heard that if you started running, and you didn't have the stress response, you'd just drop dead in about a minute or two, because your body has to do all this to get the blood flowing and enough oxygen to all your muscles. So again, in the short term, this is a good thing survival-wise. Thousands of years ago, if you were running on the savanna from a lion, the lion would get tired after a couple of minutes and then lay down. Maybe he'll try again on somebody else later. Then you would lay down in the grass, or up in a tree, and your parasympathetic response kicks in and calms you down. You realize it's over, everything is okay now, you survived that encounter, and you relax.

But today, many of us chronically feel stressed. Instead of an actual lion, it may be a mental lion. Thoughts about a deadline, or "I gotta do a good job on this report for the boss." Or your kids need something, or you're short on money, or the traffic is bad when you're late for work. Your brain can't really tell the difference between an actual lion and these kinds of mental events, so it releases the same stress chemicals to spark a survival response, though on a smaller scale.

So this short-term response leads to long-term problems. Chronically shutting down the digestive system leads to problems in your gut like ulcers or irritable bowel syndrome. Pumping your heart harder and faster can eventually lead to chronic higher blood pressure and heart problems. We have frequent tense muscles and headaches. So that's where we get into trouble—having this constant feeling of stress.

Now those of you here today look pretty calm at the moment. In some of the groups I've had, even just to sit still for our first class was a challenge for some people, because they came in with a constant urge to "do something." When standing in line, instead of just waiting, they had to pull out their phones and "accomplish something." And you know, we can relate to that when we have busy lives. But you can imagine what that does to your body if you can't even choose to sit still without this constant urge to rush around. It's this constant blast of cortisol that really does long-term damage to your body. There are different statistics on this, but research shows that up to 90% of the conditions that bring someone to a physician have some stress-related component to them.

Now it's important to know that stress by itself doesn't cause disease. It's not like when you're stressed, some disease just materializes out of the ether. One of the things it does is make you more vulnerable to disease. It messes with your immune system. In fact, in the short term, your immune system is stronger when you are under stress. Evolutionarily speaking, if you get clawed by a lion, and your guts are hanging out and dragging on the ground, your immune system kicks up to prevent infection. Have you ever had the experience of really pushing yourself at work or school for some stressful deadline, then ending up sick when you're on break or take a vacation? When the stress is gone, the immune system goes way down after being so overwhelmed. Also, with chronic stress, this hyperactive immune response can lead to autoimmune diseases, where your immune system is so active it starts eating your own body's cells.

The other thing stress does is make current conditions worse. If you already suffer from something, stress can often add additional problems and keep your body from healing itself in the best way that it can. So that's why stress affects so many different health conditions.

Any questions or thoughts on the stress response before we shift a little bit?

Before we talk about mindfulness, I thought it would be interesting to share this. It came from a collection of scientists in Europe called the New Economics Foundation (2008). They created a task force to ask what contributes to having a sense of well-being, to feeling good, instead of just focusing on disease and what's wrong. They came up with five important areas, and mindfulness relates pretty well to all of these.

The first one is "connect," connecting with people. Having family, friends, colleagues, neighbors. Interestingly, as a psychologist, it's pretty rare for someone to come in and see me that has really, really awful lifelong depression but has fantastic friendships and lots and lots of really close friends. Obviously anybody can get depressed given difficult circumstances, but people tend to rebound better if they've got good friends. If you've had really close friendships, you know they can provide a lot of support and fulfillment.

"Be active." Being active is obviously important. I think this culture often rewards the intellectual, thinking part of who we are. I'm an academic, so I do a lot of thinking, but many of us too often neglect our bodies, as if we're just this head floating around with thoughts. We've got all these other aspects of who we are. And of course, from a health perspective, exercising, and being active in the sense of getting out into the world, contributes to feeling good.

"Taking notice." This area relates the most to mindfulness, the ability to take notice, pay attention, and to be curious about life.

As we're going to talk about, mindfulness helps us step out of our habitual "automatic pilot" kind of mode. We do a lot of things automatically, out of routine, right? Have you ever been driving somewhere, and suddenly, you're magically at your home? You don't even really remember quite how you got there. Or worse yet, you were supposed to pick up somebody, and you just automatically went to your home. Doing things automatically can be helpful, in the sense that there are way too many things to have to pay attention to all the time. But if we're living our lives on this automatic pilot, always jumping to the next thing, not even noticing what we're experiencing, then we miss out on much of our lives.

Alan Watts is one of my favorite philosophers. He talks about the trick that's played on us as kids. We're always given the impression that the "good things" in life are out there somewhere, and will be coming in the future. Right? So when you're growing up, you just can't wait till you get to go to kindergarten. And then you'll get to get into first grade, then second grade, then middle school, then high school, then college. And then you'll get a job, and won't that be great? Then you'll get money, then you'll get a house, then save for a bigger house. Then you'll look forward to getting a promotion, and then you'll be able to save for retirement. We're led to believe that we'll be happy after we get something out there in the future. Then one day we wake up, often in middle age, and say, "Well, I guess I've arrived!" Instead of enjoying life as we went along, we kept postponing things. So mindfulness is about coming back to what you are experiencing right now, being more fully in the moments you are in. Obviously you need to think about the past and the future, but if you're living in thoughts all the time, you're going to end up missing most of your life. Taking notice involves catching more of the little things that are going on, fostering more appreciation of what you are currently experiencing.

I had the opportunity to spend six weeks in India and Nepal, and people prepared me for the culture shock of going there, but no one really prepared me for the culture shock of coming back. Not to stereotype, but I was in some of the poorest regions, so I just felt amazed by how clean and new everything looked when I got back home. I could drink the water whenever I wanted to, and not have to wonder whether my food had been washed with tap water. I developed more appreciation for all the little things I had taken for granted for so long. So we'll talk more about that in a few minutes.

"Keep learning." Being able to have that fresh perspective on the world. There's been a lot of research showing the more new things you do, the more brain connections you develop. We are never too old to grow brain connections. Trying new things and breaking out of old routines fosters more well-being.

And of course, "giving." Sharing with others, especially people you really care about, and your community, in whatever ways that work well for you, contributes to a sense of well-being.

So those are the five ways to well-being (New Economics Foundation, 2008), which I thought would be an interesting framework to start with.

Now, what is mindfulness? The word itself of course is common in the English language, as when I said I'd be mindful of the volume of my voice. But here we're going to use it in a pretty specific way, for developing a set of skills. Now, the thing I really want to make clear right away is that I don't have some secret. We're going to be doing some exercises, but you're going to be reawakening something that already is a natural human process. Kids are really good at just being in the moment, paying attention to details, and noticing what's happening, instead of always being stuck in thinking. So it's important to recognize that this isn't something new or artificial.

Mindfulness has been present in a lot of different cultures historically. The traditions I know the most about, which have informed some of the research, came from Asia, originating from a man named Siddhartha Gautama. He later became known as the Buddha, which just means "the person who woke up." If the average person is sort of sleepwalking through life on automatic pilot, this is somebody who woke up to the moment. When Siddhartha became keenly aware that life is short, and of all the suffering in the world, he decided to go on a quest for answers.

Siddhartha's teachers at the time taught a practice known as "absorption meditation," which is a very blissful state. People will describe it as feeling "one with the universe." Interestingly, researchers put people practicing this kind of meditation into brain scanners (Newberg, D'Aquili, & Rause, 2001). There's a part of your brain called the orientation association area, in the parietal lobe. One side tells you, "This is outside me, this is not me, that's outside my body." The other side of your brain tells you, "This is me, this is my space, my body." Babies don't have that same sense until their brains develop more fully, so they'll just grab onto anything. These brain scans found that the activity levels drop in these areas, so you literally can't feel the difference between your body and what's not your body. So when they say, "I feel one with the universe," it's a literal, subjective description, because they don't feel any separation from what's inside and outside their bodies.

The problem with only doing that type of practice is, once you get up off the meditation cushion, back to reality, nothing has really changed in the world. It's valuable for relaxing, feeling refreshed, and getting a broader perspective, but you are likely to find all the same problems with your life and personality that you had before. It is wonderful to go off into this blissful state, but it doesn't always apply so much in daily life. One of Siddhartha's contributions was to develop a systematic method of training the mind called *sati*, or *vipassana*, known as insight, or mindfulness.

The research on mindfulness is booming so fast, it's hard to keep up with it. They've taken people through an eight-week group, like the one we offer here, and scanned their brains before and after. They actually found changes in the physical structure of the brain, in areas related to things like emotion regulation, sense of self, and short-term memory (Lazar et al., 2005).

Again, feel free to jump in at any time with questions or comments, because I get excited about this topic, so I'll just keep going and going.

There are many definitions of mindfulness, but my favorite is from Jon Kabat-Zinn. Has anybody read any of his books, or seen any of his lectures? He's really one of the pioneers, who took these techniques and systematized them into a program that was reproducible, and could undergo scientific scrutiny. He defines it as, "The awareness that emerges through paying attention, on purpose, in the present moment, non-judgmentally, to the unfolding of experience from moment to moment" (Kabat-Zinn, 2003, p. 145).

Let's break this down. "Awareness that emerges" is that waking up I was talking about—just noticing that you are noticing, being able to suddenly choose what you want to pay attention to. Take your feet, for example. Chances are you had no conscious thought of your feet a moment ago. But you might choose to notice, how do my feet feel? Maybe you don't feel anything in particular. Maybe they're hurting. Maybe you choose what you want to pay attention to next. Suddenly you're consciously choosing. That's the "on purpose" part of the definition. I'm consciously choosing. Mindfulness is a very conscious, intentional process. I choose what to pay more attention to.

"Paying attention" is the vehicle of mindfulness. There are several different kinds of attention from a brain perspective (Posner & Rafal, 1986; Sohlberg & Mateer, 1989). There's being able to focus on something, sustaining your attention on something, choosing to ignore a lot of other things that are going on around the room, and being able to let go of something and shift your attention to another something. There's also divided attention, but most of us practice that a lot already, like when you're driving, eating, and talking on the phone at the same time. Each of these types of attention has a different brain pathway, and the more you practice, the stronger the brain connections get. This is a lot like physical exercise. The more you lift weights, the more your muscles grow, and the more you can lift. The more you practice paying attention, the stronger those circuits become in your brain, and the easier it gets over time. And like physical exercise, it's not enough to just understand how it works, or just do it a few times. You have to practice regularly.

The next part is "in the present moment." That means being able to keep coming back to what I am experiencing right now. It's a gift that our brains have the ability to think about other times, right? If I can anticipate what might happen, I can prepare for it, and then might live longer and reproduce more. If I remember the past, I can learn better how to survive. But very often we get stuck living in the future and the past more than we're living in the present. Mindfulness is about coming back, over and over again, to this moment.

Now, many people find the next part, "non-judgmentally," to be the hardest. What that means is choosing to at least temporarily let go of that compulsive tendency of the brain to make comparisons all the time. Instead of enjoying the friend you're talking with, you might be thinking, "Well my other friend is so much nicer. I should've spent time with them! What am I doing here?" Judgments can be very good things, and you may very well choose to say goodbye to your friend and go somewhere else if they are being very negative. But when you're constantly making comparisons, you are in your head, and not experiencing what is actually happening in the moment as much. Very often, we compulsively judge ourselves, berating ourselves for not being good enough, or for not doing something right. Even in mindfulness practice, you may notice yourself thinking, "I'm so distracted, why can't I do this right? Oh no, I'm judging myself! Oh darn it, now I'm judging my judgment of myself!" Mindfulness involves just noticing what is happening. "I'm having trouble concentrating right now," or "Judgments are here," and bringing your awareness back to where you want it, over and over again.

And the last part is "to the unfolding of experience from moment to moment," which refers to the active, dynamic aspect of mindfulness. It's not just sitting still, it's bringing it into your life. Now in class, we will do some exercises where we just sit still. It's much like exercising, where you stand still and move weights back and forth. We're practicing to build up our "mental muscles" in here. But the goal is to bring it into your life. It's not much use to only be present when you're sitting alone quietly in a room. You want to bring it into your relationships, and into your work, and into your interactions with the world around you. In the groups, we do some exercises with movement, and also practice bringing it into daily activities. One of the assignments we ask people to do is to pay more attention to one routine activity per day that they're already doing, like brushing their teeth. Have you ever been in such a hurry that you walked out the door in the morning, then you stopped to think, "I can't remember, did I even brush my teeth this morning? I not sure if I can taste it—I better go do it again." You were doing it quickly and automatically. We just ask people to slow it down, and to notice all the things going on. The feel of the knob, the squeaking sounds as it turns, the smell of the water wafting up, the sparkle of the water as it splatters and runs down the drain. Noticing the subtle muscle coordination it takes to put the brush under the water, which hits the bristles with a little bit of pressure. There's really a lot going on. That doesn't necessarily mean that brushing your teeth has to become a mystical experience, but it's a way of practicing more often, and noticing more about things as they are.

So how does mindfulness actually work? Here's the reason why this has caught so much scientific attention. Obviously it's been around thousands of years, and the people who have been doing this didn't need to wait for scientists to tell them it works, but putting it into scientific language helped researchers to see what's really going on, and how it can help with modern problems.

Let's start with how thinking can get us into trouble. We're very reliant on thinking. Of course, thinking is good—you don't want to stop thinking. But we get overreliant on it for fixing problems. Earlier, I was having some trouble getting the computer projector to come up, so I starting thinking about it, pushed the right button, and then magically the screen popped up. So that rewarded my thinking. Thinking got me what I needed. But too often we try to use thinking to "fix" our thinking or "fix" our feelings. If we don't like the way that we're feeling, we start thinking to try and fix our feelings. If it's something in the past, we go over and over it—"I should have done this differently," "I wish I would have said that," or "I wish this could have been different." We can also get stuck in the future, worried about all the things that *might* happen.

In a sense, we can become addicted to our thinking. While I'm thinking about fixing my feelings and my thoughts, I'm in my head, so I don't feel them in my body as much. If I'm feeling anxious or stressed, and I start thinking, while I'm thinking, I'm not feeling it as much, so my experience of that bad feeling goes down a little bit.

Sorry if I'm slipping into professor mode here. Ask me questions as we go along if any of this doesn't make sense. It took me a little while to wrap my head fully around this.

Because by definition we don't like unpleasant feelings, if something makes a bad feeling go down, our brains are wired to say, "Whatever you just did, it was working—do more of that." That's why addictions are such big problems, because when you take a drink of alcohol, your bad feelings go down, and your brain can develop an urge to keep doing that when the bad feelings come back up again. So in a funny way, you get addicted to thinking. You try to out-think your feelings. But you know, you can't out-think a feeling. A feeling is a feeling. But while you're thinking, you're not feeling as much. Thinking is distracting you, so the bad feeling goes down, which makes you want to keep thinking.

Now, for all the grey areas in psychology, anxiety is one of the things we understand the most. Let's say you came to me with a phobia of water bottles. Maybe when you gave a presentation, somebody got upset and hit you in the head with a green water bottle like this one. So when you see this green water bottle, your brain remembers when you got hit with one, and you have this awful feeling of the circumstances and how embarrassed you felt. You might step away from the water bottle, and when you do that, you feel a little bit better, because now it's farther away. So, over time, you literally develop this habit—whenever you see one or get near one, you feel bad, so you back away from it and feel better. That's how phobias develop. Over time, your attempts to avoid feeling anxious can become so strong that you won't get near something you're afraid of, or don't want to even say the word. You can spend a lot of energy trying not to think about something.

The treatment for this type of anxiety is really effective. We expose people to the object they are afraid of, or have them repeat the word, or they look at pictures. When the anxiety comes up, instead of backing away or avoiding it, they just feel it. When you can't escape, you may think you're going to die. When you stay with it, it will often get even worse at first. But if you just stay there, and wait long enough, the anxiety always comes back down. It's just physiologically how the brain is wired. After it comes down, you can then move a little closer to what you fear. The anxiety will jump right back up again, but you remember what happened the last time, and you wait it out. It'll get a little worse at first, but it will get better if you stay with it. Eventually, you're able to hug and kiss the water bottle, or whatever it was you were compulsively avoiding. You've rewired your brain.

Here's how this helps with stress. When I become stressed, instead of constantly worrying and thinking about it, I can let myself feel my body. I feel the stress in my heart, my stomach, my throat, wherever it is. It feels a little worse at first, because I'm opening myself up to it, but it always levels off and comes back down. And here's the thing—once the body sensations go down, I've got less pressure to distract myself with thoughts. The worries and ruminations lose their fuel. People I work with talk so much about how free their minds become, because they've been spending so many hours of every day habitually thinking about stuff that they can't control. Once that pressure is gone, they can think about what they want to think about, and are more open to just experiencing the pleasurable things in their daily lives. They also become more clear and conscious about how they work with the negative things. That's what is fascinating to me about mindfulness—it's not just a tool for working with problems, but it helps you appreciate all the small things in life as well.

Another thing that's going on is a process called "defusion" or "decentering," which is about changing our relationship to our thoughts. We often get "fused," or overidentified, with our thinking. If you struggle with depression, you might commonly have thoughts like, "I'm worthless. I can't do anything right. I'm no good." You feel like those thoughts are who you are. This may sound like semantics, but what can happen is that you start to recognize, "Oh, I'm having a thought that 'I am no good,' that must mean I'm getting depressed. I better go do something to take care of myself." Instead of arguing with your own thoughts, and getting caught up in them, you can get perspective on what you're thinking, what you're feeling, and what you're experiencing. Getting some distance allows you more conscious choice in how to respond to what's going on.

As I mentioned, developing this as a reliable skill requires some systematic training, which is the purpose of the eight-week program. It helps to have a group of other people going through this with you, for motivation and for learning from each other's experiences.

It is important to talk about how mindfulness is different from other methods. The first one, absorption meditation, I talked about earlier. Hypnosis can a very useful tool, which involves suspending your conscious mind and communicating with your subconscious mind. In contrast, mindfulness is about increasing your conscious awareness. It is about paying more attention and becoming more alert.

Because we often experience stress, relaxation is very important. However, mindfulness is not necessarily meant to relax you. It may sound funny, but relaxation is more of a side effect of being more present with what's going on. It often happens when you stop fighting your own experiences. You can't "force" yourself to relax. If you are anxious in this moment, you can't make yourself feel relaxed about it. But if you allow yourself to feel the anxiety, and let go of the struggle with it, it is more likely to pass naturally.

The ironic thing about relaxation methods is that they sometimes make stress worse, especially if they are used to avoid dealing with something. It's like taking a vacation. Have you ever had this experience? Assuming you can forget about work while you're on vacation, typically when you come back, all the work you should have been doing while you were gone has piled up on top of your usual workload. You're thrown right back into it, and almost in a shocking kind of way for some people, depending on how much you like your job.

A similar type of thing can happen with relaxation methods if they're used for avoidance. If you don't like the stress of what's going on in the moment, you might try to escape it by thinking about being at the beach. And then when you're thrown back into it, you may feel worse than you did before. Now relaxation is very important. It helps your body recover and recuperate, and that part of it is very healing. But if that is the only tool you have for dealing with stress, it won't be helpful in the midst of difficult situations. Mindfulness is more about moving right into the middle what is happening, and working with your thoughts, feelings, and sensations as they come up instead of just avoiding them. Amazingly, you can develop more calm presence even within the busiest days.

There are quite a few mental health programs now that incorporate mindfulness. A number of them now have enough research to be considered evidenced-based practices, which is considered a pretty huge deal in the health care field. These aren't just ideas about what might work—these programs have gone through randomized, controlled research trials to show their effectiveness.

So, you've all managed to stay awake as I've been yapping on and on [laughter]. Any questions or thoughts before we do a 3-minute exercise, to give you a taste of what this is like?

[Exercise—3-minute breathing space]

Anybody feel comfortable sharing anything about what that was like, or any questions about that exercise?

In a sense, this is an encapsulation of the whole program, because it contains several longer exercises that we practice in the course, but this allows us to quickly check in with ourselves. Instead of letting things build up all day, we practice tuning in more often, which helps interrupt the negative cycles we can get into. For example, very rarely will a headache just pop up out of nowhere. It might start with some back tension, that leads to some shoulder tension, that leads to some neck tension, that builds up throughout the day without our awareness. Just checking in and taking a breath tends to interrupt that buildup. It also kicks in our parasympathetic relaxation response that counters stress.

I had a meditation teacher once say, "Your homework assignment is to breathe six times a day." Of course, we all laughed. "We breathe thousands of times a day, what are you talking about?" But try it sometime. If you can just remember to stop at various times throughout the day and take a breath, you'll be amazed at how much it can short circuit any tension and stress that might build up. A lot of my students have found programs for their phones that you can set to go off at random times, as a reminder to pause, take a breath, and check into the moment. One student told me she found herself really looking forward to when that bell was going to go off. Of course, I laughingly told her she could stop and take a breath whenever she wanted to.

So one of the points of this course is to bring more awareness into your daily life. More often noticing what's going on in yourself, as it is happening, allows for more conscious responses instead of automatic reactions. It's very much like the 24-hour rule with an email. Have you ever gotten a really nasty email, and you fired back and told them off, then the next day you realized you overreacted? If you have a strong reaction to an email, it may be better to wait a day before you respond.

Similarly, mindfulness can help us pause anytime we get worked up, even if only for a fraction of a second. If something really upsets you, you can see it as a sign that something important is going on, before you react in a way that might make things worse.

Now it could very well be that you have every right to be angry. Anger can motivate us to take decisive action. But if you are only reacting automatically, you could make the situation worse. Have you ever had the experience of reacting so strongly that suddenly you're the person that looks out of control or unreasonable, even though someone else was causing the whole situation? Mindfulness helps us recognize our automatic reactions.

As we get better at noticing our own thoughts, we can choose whether to investigate them or let them go. Sometimes we notice old patterns of thinking that are not helpful, and we might choose to let them go and come back into the moment. But sometimes, when the thoughts keep returning, we might choose to investigate them to see if there is something we need to learn from them.

I'll skip over this because of time, but it's a poem by Billy Collins that embodies some of the attitudes of mindfulness. Sometimes we'll share poems in the groups because they can express things that are hard to describe.

The groups that I do here follow the mindfulness-based cognitive therapy protocol. We meet for eight sessions, an hour and a half each, on Monday nights. We mainly focus on stress, which we can all relate to, but people often come in with things like depression, anxiety, chronic pain, and other problems, so we'll discuss those things as well. Our discussions are very practical about how these principles apply to real life, and I encourage direct questions and even challenges, rather than thinking that if you just do these exercises your life will magically become easy.

If you choose to come to the group, we do ask you to commit to doing about 45 minutes of home practice each day between the sessions. The idea of it is exactly like physical exercise. If you exercise regularly, you'll get a lot more benefit. Because you're overcoming years and years of automatic kinds of behaviors, it takes some time and practice. Everybody will get a CD so you can practice the exercises at home.

Are any of you health care providers by chance?

Laura: Eye doctor—optometrist.

Dr. Sears: Those of us who are providers, or parents or caregivers for that matter, are constantly attending to other people and often neglect our own needs. A study done with psychology students found that an eight-week course like the one we're doing not only reduced their negative feelings, like stress and anxiety, it also increased positive feelings, like happiness and self-esteem (Shapiro, Brown, & Biegel, 2007). Once you start letting go of all the stress and anxiety, you may begin to recognize and work with deeper issues like how you feel about yourself.

In another interesting study (Grepmair et al., 2007), they randomly assigned therapists to take training like this, and their patients had better outcomes than the therapists that didn't have the training. Isn't that a funny thing? I think one of the reasons for that could be just that sense of connection you develop from practicing mindfulness. Instead of thinking about what I should be saying, or the next patient that is coming in the door, I'm just here. I'm more present with the people I'm with. And that's powerful in and of itself. Have you ever had a provider that barely makes eye contact, and abruptly answers your questions before you even finish asking them, and rushes back out the door?

We experience this all the time on the phone, right? Have you ever been talking to somebody, and you're not even sure why, but you suddenly stop and ask "Hello? Are you there?" They may say, "Oh, yeah, I'm listening." But you just know they must have been checking their email, or doing something else. You can just tell they were not really engaged with you somehow. Mindfulness practice helps you become more consciously engaged with people when you want to be.

These are just some books I recommend if you want more background on this material. *Full Catastrophe Living* is about the original course that Jon Kabat-Zinn (2013) developed. *The Mindful Way Through Depression* (Williams, Teasdale, Segal, & Kabat-Zinn, 2007) and *The Mindful Way Workbook* (Teasdale, Williams, & Segal, 2014) were written by the developers of this course, so you can read it as you go along if you want to more fully digest the material. They also come with great CDs of mindfulness exercises. If you're interested in the clinical applications of mindfulness, I wrote a book with my friends Dennis Tirch and Robert Denton called *Mindfulness in Clinical Practice* (Sears, Tirch, & Denton, 2011).

And lastly, here is my contact info, and the number for the front desk here if you're interested in signing up for the course. Any questions or comments?

Stephanie: When you talk about the home practice, is it written homework, is it practicing what we're learning in the class, is it? . . .

Dr. Sears: I already have the handouts for the next class if you'd like to see. For each class, everybody gets a handout, which describes the theme and important concepts for the week, and describes the home practice assignments. For the first week, you do an exercise called the body scan once a day, following along with the CD I will give you. The second thing is to keep track of how the exercises are going on this sheet, which is only for your own reference—you don't have to show it to anyone. Another assignment is to practice paying more attention to one routine activity every day, to see what you notice. You will also practice paying more attention when you are eating.

Any other questions?

Laura: On the flyer it said it's important to be here for all eight classes. I'm actually going to miss the second one. I'm going to be on vacation.

Dr. Sears: A lot of people miss one or two due to life circumstances. I'm happy to email or give you copies of the handouts ahead of time. You are also welcome to call me on the phone or stay before or after another class to get a quick catch-up.

One of the nice things about this practice is that you don't really have to memorize anything. Mindfulness is a natural process you already possess, so each session is like looking at it from a different angle. It's not like learning calculus, where you're lost if you miss something. It's about getting us back to a more centered, natural state of being.

Laura: How long have you been doing this? This particular course?

Dr. Sears: Probably about five years total, but two years here.

Laura: Have you done any follow-up with people who have gone through the class, like a couple of years later, and asked if it is still making a difference for them?

Dr. Sears: Yeah, though I haven't done it systematically in the way that researchers should.

Laura: Anything anecdotal? Anybody contact you later?

Dr. Sears: Yeah, I've had both. Some people send me random emails about how much it has changed their lives. Some come back as private therapy clients to work on deeper issues. In fact, I just saw a woman earlier today who started with my mindfulness group, and I've been seeing her for four years now. It's still part of her life. I've had other people say the group was so helpful, but then life got busy, and they stopped practicing the exercises. So they came back to get a boost, to get back into that mindset again.

Christine: My concern is that I'll do great through the group, and then start to get lazy when there's no longer a class to go to.

Dr. Sears: That's a common concern, and we address it directly in the group. On the one hand, the nice thing is that all through the group, we reinforce the practice of noticing what is happening more often throughout the day. Maybe you're sitting in the car, and you notice you're grabbing the wheel very tightly, and you realize you're a little stressed. So even right then, you are practicing mindfulness, giving yourself more conscious choice in what you do next. But given how long we have practiced doing things automatically, we'll talk about ways to personalize and keep up regular practice. I'll also be offering regular "booster sessions" where you can come in and reconnect with the practice, compare notes with others, and learn some other exercises.

Any more questions?

Laura: How large is a typical group?

Dr. Sears: It varies. I've had as few as three. The last one I had here was 19. I think just a few people signed up this time.

Laura: Is this where we'll meet?

Dr. Sears: Yes, it'll be in this room. Anything else?

Stephanie: Can I get a copy of the PowerPoint?

Dr. Sears: Sure—I actually have one here that you can have. And you all have my number and email if you have any other questions. If that's it, I'll see you next week!

5 Session 1

Awareness and Autopilot

The first MBCT session introduces mindfulness in a concrete and practical way. It is about bringing awareness to things that we normally do automatically. The raisin exercise engages all of our senses as we pay attention to the process of eating. The body scan is used to systematically and purposefully move our attention throughout the entire body. These exercises are very simple but can also be difficult to do, which teaches us about how our minds operate.

In this first session, it is important to give informed consent, clarifying such things as the nature of the group (educational versus traditional psychotherapy) and issues of confidentiality.

Since this group was small, I had each of them introduce themselves to the entire group. Ideally, the participants should break into dyads first. I find people chat much more this way and feel more connected to at least one other person in the group.

The second edition also suggests setting aside a few minutes toward the end of the session to discuss potential obstacles and how to deal with them, since many participants have challenges in getting a regular practice started (Segal, Williams, & Teasdale, 2013).

Of note, I find that a casual atmosphere works best. If people come early and there seems to be an awkward silence, I let them know it is okay to talk before the session begins.

In this class, Kevin took his shoes off at the beginning, which emitted a strong odor. As the session went on, I had an internal debate about whether or not to say something in front of the others. Ignoring such a strong stimulus was not modeling mindfulness, but I also didn't want to embarrass someone who was struggling with a lot of anxiety. As it happened, he approached me after class, so I had a chance to mention this to him in private. He apologized, admitting that he had been working out before class. He was accustomed to taking his shoes off to show respect from his years of living in Asia. I let him know everyone could keep their shoes on since we sat in chairs.

You will also notice a couple of participants in this session with strong emotions—one felt so much anxiety he wanted to run out of the room, and one was crying during the class. Rather than falling into therapist mode to "fix" these emotions, it is important to model staying present with them.

Session 1 Transcript

Dr. Sears: Welcome everyone! First of all, I salute you for making the commitment to yourself to come here. I know it's not always easy to make time for self-care.

Before we get started, it's important to talk about confidentiality. Even though I promote this as a class, by profession I am a psychologist and therapist. According to my ethics code, I have to always live up to the highest standard, which is to keep things confidential, and to not divulge anything personal that goes on in the group, with certain exceptions like imminent danger of harm. And of course, I ask every one of you here in the group to keep things confidential. What goes on here should stay here. Now obviously, I can't guarantee that other people will keep full confidentiality, so if you have some super critical, secret information, you might not want to share that with the entire group.

As I mentioned in the intro, this is not intended to be a psychotherapy group in the sense of delving into the past, or getting into deeply personal issues. Our purpose is to learn and apply mindfulness skills. If things do come up, you're welcome to share at the level you're comfortable with, as it relates to the course material. For example, someone might share, "During the week, I was with my partner, and we began arguing. I recognized how tense I was getting, and so I took a couple of breaths and noticed how I was feeling. I was then able to continue talking a little more, and we were able to work it through. Usually, we would have gotten into a big fight and gone for days without talking." So, talking about how it's working for you, and what's not working for you, which I think is helpful to integrate the skills into your life. But it's up to you. You could literally go through the entire group and not say a word, though you will get a lot more out of this course if you actively participate.

I also find challenging questions are often the most important. I've been in some groups where you're not supposed to challenge the teacher, but I enjoy a good challenge. This group is not about imitating me, or being worthy of getting something from me. It's about making it practical and useful in your own life. It's about becoming more fully yourself.

Any questions or comments about any of that?

It may be helpful to just quickly get a sense of what everybody is here for. Maybe just your first name, in the way of an introduction, and of course you don't have to give any details unless you

	want to. I like to customize things a little for the people in the group, so it helps me to hear what you are hoping to get, even if it's just, "less stress," or "my doctor told me to come and I don't know why I'm here." Also, if you have any particular background in mindfulness, or another meditation practice, you can share that if you like. So, first name, what you're hoping to get out of this, and any background you want to mention.
Stephanie:	I'm Stephanie. I actually took Tai Chi for seven years, and I still take it, though not on a regular basis. I kinda got out of the habit of meditating, because my mind always wandered. I'm going through a divorce, and I think I can benefit from some stress reduction, and working through some sadness.
Dr. Sears:	Thank you.
Laura:	I'm Laura. I've always been kind of a nervous person, like when I'm in new situations and that sort of thing. But the past couple of years, I feel like I have this constant underlying anxiety. But it's not anything specific. So I kind of want to get that under control. That's about it. Oh, and I have some hearing loss, so if you could talk a little louder that would be great.
Dr. Sears:	Oh, okay. I apologize. You did tell me that already. I do tend to talk softly. I'll work on that.
Christine:	I'm Christine. I have some involved health problems that go back to when I was young. I have Cushing's disease, which causes your cortisol levels to go pretty high and to stay that way for periods of time, which is like you're under extra stress all the time. I'm being treated for that, but it's not completely under control. I also have a seizure disorder, which makes it hard to keep my nervous system calm as much as I'd like. So, that's why I'm here.
Kevin:	We'd like our cortisol levels to be what? Is it better if they're lower, or higher, or what?
Christine:	It changes. Low or high is fine, but if you're high all the time, it wears your body down.
Dr. Sears:	Yeah. It's about balance. Thank you.
Kim:	I'm Kim. And right now I don't work. I'm a single mom with three boys, from 16 years to 20 months. My oldest two both have mental health challenges. My oldest has autism. So it's very stressful at home, and I myself am dealing with chronic illness that is not responding to medications anymore, and I'm in a lot of pain, and stress all the time. I started doing meditation on Sundays at church and found it helpful. I talked to Dr. Tiffany about it, and she recommended this class. She thought this might help me where medications can't.
Dr. Sears:	Welcome.
Kevin:	I'm Kevin. I was raised mostly around here, but have spent the last 12 years in Asia. I'm back here mostly because I wanted to spend

some time with my parents, who are aging. While I was here visiting, my mother had a fall, and so she needs some extra caretaking. My father's 87, and has been doing all the caretaking, so that's a lot on him. They are in a retirement community, so there is support around, but you have to call for it and ask for it. I tried meditation years ago—I used to go to the local Zen center sometimes with my brother. And like you were saying, when I try to meditate, it ends up being an experience more in frustration than redemption, because my mind is jumping all over so much I can't control it. I try to just observe it, "Okay, let it come, let it go," but it keeps coming and going to the point where I'm like, "You know what, I know my mind is jumping all over the place. I'd rather be playing tennis—at least I can focus on the ball or something!" [laughter]. So I haven't had real good success with sitting meditation. I do it in other ways. I do some yoga now, and it works for me. My immediate challenge is I stopped using an antidepressant medication six months ago that I had been on for many years. There's a lot of depression in my family history, so it's kind of stacked against me. But I had this healthy lifestyle, and I decided, no more synthetic meds for me. So I stopped gradually. Since then, it's been rough, really rough, because now I'm confronting whatever the original condition was that I had to be on those things in the first place. So, I have daily, strong, strong anxiety. I'm actually controlling my anxiety with Ambien, which is what most people take for sleep, but fortunately for me, I have high energy levels, and Ambien doesn't make me drowsy during the day. So that's kind of what keeps me coherent, gets me through the day, until we find out the bigger picture, what's out of balance. So, anxiety and unpredictable crying spells, which can be pretty intense.

Dr. Sears: Glad you're here. Thanks, everybody. Even in this very initial piece, I appreciate your courage in sharing what brought you in here. And it's obvious too, as we listen to each other, this is serious stuff. We're not talking about a little more calming. All of you, in your own way, are going through some pretty significant things. So I'm happy to say we'll be addressing the things you're working on in a very real way. In my experience, both in doing these groups and clinically, this works well for all of the things you're talking about. Not in the sense that magically everything goes away, and becomes all sweetness and light, but in giving you a tool for working with these things.

So it's not going to be just, "Get more sleep, and eat right, and try to think happy thoughts!" I'm poking fun a little bit, but I mean to say that we're not going to ignore your very real problems—we're really going to jump right into the middle of them. Sleep and diet are of course very important, and they often get disrupted by stress, anxiety, and depression. But we're also going to explore all those things your mind is doing, and we'll come to notice that often the ways that we're trying to fix our stress are the very things that contribute to keeping it going. We're going to be talking about those patterns that we get stuck in accidentally.

I joke about the happy thoughts, but interestingly, there is some research that if you try to make yourself think happy thoughts, sometimes you feel worse. A part of your mind knows that what you're saying isn't true in the moment, highlighting the separation between where you are now and where you want to be. But wherever we are is where we are, so that's where we have to start from.

Alan Watts tells a story about a man who was lost in the countryside in England. He finally went up to a local and asked how to get to the town he was looking for. The local scratched his head and said, "Well sir, I do know the way, but if I were you, I wouldn't start from here!" You know, it's a silly joke, but the truth of it is, we feel that way all the time. Here's where I am, but I don't like where I am, I want to be somewhere else. When I'm courageous, then I'll get some courage. Or when I'm full of love, then I'll be loving. Or when I don't feel anxiety, then I'll be happy. But before I can get anywhere, I have to acknowledge where I am, and what I'm starting with.

That's the acceptance piece of mindfulness that we'll be talking about. It doesn't mean I have to like it. It doesn't have to be a feeling of resignation. It's just recognizing that like it or not, deserve it or not, here is where I am. I have to start from here. If I can accept that this is what I got, that this is the way it is right now, then I can let go of my struggle and my resistance to it. And then I can more easily move toward something more important to me.

I may be jumping ahead a little bit with all of that, but I want to emphasize right away that we can all be real in here. And by the way, if you've got back or pain issues, feel free to stand up, or sit however you feel comfortable. If we're meditating and you need to shift your body, feel free. I was joking earlier about some other meditation places I've been to, where if your back pops or something, everybody stares at you.

Kevin: You moved!

Dr. Sears: Yeah. I just want to make it clear that it's okay to be yourself, shift your body, or do whatever you need to. Now, I might make some suggestions for you. For instance, sometimes avoiding something makes it worse, so if you're feeling a little anxiety, and you feel like you really need to leave the room, you could certainly go ahead and leave, but you might experiment with allowing yourself to feel it for a little while first, and then decide. I haven't driven anybody from the room yet [laughter], but that's a possibility, so I want you to feel safe enough to let me know about that. And obviously, anytime you need to go to the bathroom, feel free to go.

Kevin: Do you think we should vocalize that, or just keep it internal—that kind of dialogue, monologue—of the thinking, (whispering) "God, I think I might need to leave the room right now!"

Dr. Sears: We're always going to process what we notice after an exercise, asking, "What was that like?", "How did that work for you?", "What was going on for you?", and you're welcome to share at that point. If you do leave the room, it would be good to let someone know if you'll be back.

Before we go on intellectually, let's start with the first exercise, unless anyone has any questions or thoughts so far. I really want to give you more of an experience before we talk more about mindfulness. Our first exercise is going to involve eating.

[Does Raisin Exercise]

Dr. Sears: So what did people notice? What sensations were present? What was your experience during that? Just at a very concrete level, what did you notice?

Christine: It's really hard to chew slowly.

Dr. Sears: Uh-huh. You noticed an urge to chew more quickly?

Christine: Yeah.

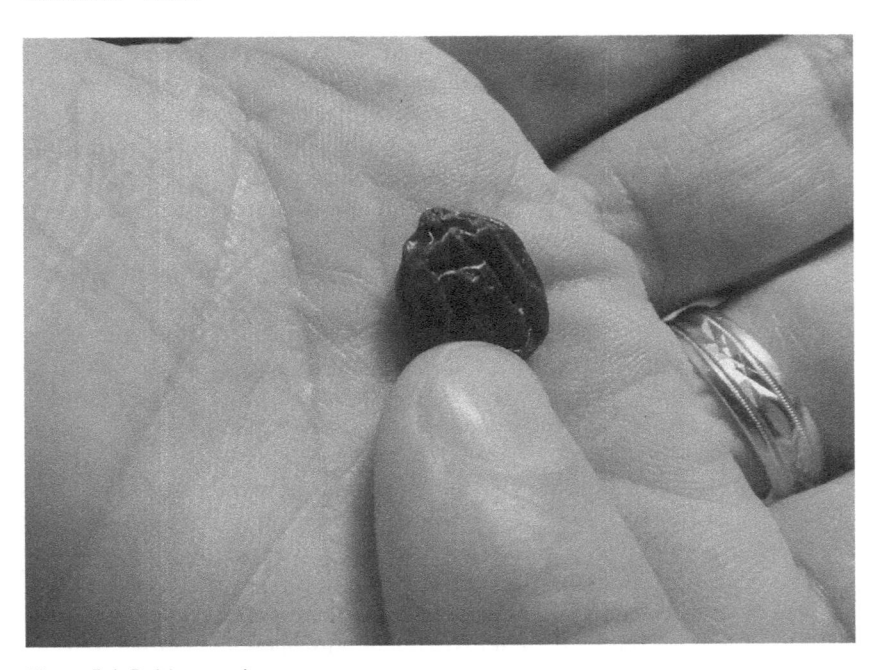

Figure 5.1 Raisin exercise

Kevin:	I had associations with little rabbit or other animal pellets out in the woods, running on trails when I was a kid in the woods. Size and texture-wise.
Dr. Sears:	Okay. So you had some memories pop up. Anybody else have memories come up? [affirmative nods] And were you able to come back to what was right here?
Kevin:	Yeah.
Kim:	I don't like raisins. So I had to focus on just what the texture was, and what the smell was, and not, "I don't like it, I don't like it, I don't like it." I did notice myself focusing on exactly what you were telling us to do, pushing that other stuff back.
Dr. Sears:	Yeah. Good. That's really important, because mindfulness is not about, "Oh, everything's peace and light." I mean, that can be a nice side effect, and it does happen, but the reality of life is that we encounter things we don't like, that we don't want. And how do we relate to that? How do we handle it? So, you were able to just keep coming back to the sensations, even though your mind was like, "I don't like this. I hope I don't have to eat this!" Did you decide not to put it in your mouth?
Kim:	I kept it under my tongue. I tried.
Dr. Sears:	Wow. Okay. So you tried a different experience. Even if you didn't put it in your mouth, you're just noticing, "Oh, that's the choice I made. I'm aware of what I'm experiencing." So that's great. So you were feeling a kind of resistance in your body? Or thoughts?
Kim:	Thoughts. Yeah. It wasn't even my body. I thought, "I'm going to just swallow it like a pill." My head was just like, "You don't like it. You don't like these. You don't like the aftertaste." So I just kept it under my tongue.
Dr. Sears:	Okay. Good. What did others notice?
Stephanie:	I think just being in the present moment, I was just aware of sadness. And I think, just putting my focus on something in this room just brought about that sadness. And then I was like, "Hell, it's just a raisin—no need to get all emotional about it!" [laughter]. And then I realized, I was just like, "Wow—that's what being in the present moment can help me do!" It's being in touch with what I'm dealing with. And when I put it in my mouth, I was aware of all the saliva that came. That's an involuntary reaction, but my mouth had seemed like it was dry, so as soon as I put the raisin in my mouth, just all this saliva. So my mouth was crying too, I guess [laughter].
Dr. Sears:	Yeah. So you were noticing as you were doing it that the sadness was just here. You weren't distracting yourself. It was here, it was here.
Stephanie:	Yeah. Exactly. So if I cry a lot, I'm okay, I'm just sad about something. But what I've also found out is whenever I cry, that's also just letting my sadness be, and release.

Dr. Sears: Yeah. Anything else anybody wants to share about what they noticed?

So typically we'll explore three questions after these exercises. The first one is just, "What did you notice?", which helps us start to disentangle all the sense experiences, feelings, memories, and thoughts. "I noticed this is what I was thinking. I noticed this feeling was present. I noticed the light shining in a certain way. I noticed this made a little crackling sound." And by the way, I used to say, "Hold it by your ear and see if it makes a sound," but a couple of people said, "I was holding the raisin by my ear, and I couldn't hear a thing!" So now I remember to say, "roll it between your fingers" [laughter]. At least for me, it makes a little snap, crackle, pop kind of sound.

Kevin: I put it too close to my ear, and then I didn't want to eat it [laughter].

Dr. Sears: Good to notice! [laughter]. But see, our experiences, our difficulties, especially for things like pain, are so intermixed with so many different things. We're just starting to break it apart a little bit. What do you notice? What do you see, what do you feel, what do you hear, smell, and taste, in this moment, as it's happening?

So the second question I ask is, how is this different from the way you might normally do whatever the exercise is, in this case, eating? How is this different, if at all, from the way you would normally eat your food?

Stephanie: It's very different. All the concentration, the focus. Even the saliva, being aware of that. I don't eat very mindfully, and I didn't realize that until we did that exercise.

Dr. Sears: Yeah.

Kevin: Well for people who have anxiety as a struggle, although I know it's really good to sit down and have a slow, calm meal and chew thoroughly, the reality is, 90% of the time it's not an option for me these days, because of the anxiety.

Dr. Sears: Let me say that another way. For you, you'd rather eat quickly than risk feeling the anxiety?

Kevin: Mmmm. Yeah. I feel like I can't sit down and join my parents at the table. It's too antsy. It's just too uncomfortable. So it's more comfortable to eat standing.

Dr. Sears: Okay. Yeah. So normally, like you said, we're just kind of on this automatic pilot. Have you ever done this before: maybe you're watching TV or talking with a friend, and then you look down and all your food's gone, and so you go get more, because you didn't really taste it. It's just changing the quality of awareness. Now actually, you don't have to eat that slowly, right? You know, if you ate your whole meal like we just ate that raisin, it would take three hours. But it's just noticing and being more conscious.

Session 1: Awareness and Autopilot 71

The theme for today is automatic pilot. Recognizing how often we do things automatically, without noticing. And as we talked about last week, that can be a really good thing sometimes, because the world is so complicated, we can't pay attention constantly to every little thing. It would be burdensome to always ask yourself, "Do I put my foot here like this, or like this, or like this?" You just kind of walk automatically. But we can get into trouble when our automatic ways of dealing with things are not helpful anymore. Maybe we learned them in the past for an extreme situation, and they just don't fit so much now. I had five siblings, so I remember that at dinner time, I had to eat fast so I could get all the food I wanted. It became a pattern. At the time, it helped me get more food. But as I got older, I'd be sitting there eating with somebody, and they'd just be starting on their second bite, and I'd look down and all my food would be gone. So recognizing, "Oh, I don't have to do that anymore."

So the next question is, "What in the heck does eating a raisin the way we just did have anything to do with why we're here—dealing with stress, pain, anxiety, depression, or whatever it is? What can we learn from an exercise like this, or what might it have to do with the reason we're all here? There's no one perfect answer—what do you think?

Kevin: To get us outside of our brains. To get us outside of our minds, and our ruminating thoughts, and to redirect them to the senses, and something else out of ourselves.

Dr. Sears: Yeah. Yeah. Absolutely. You bring up an important point—that there are two ways of knowing: thinking and experiencing. Many of you noticed that your thoughts about this exercise were very different from what you experienced through your senses.

Laura: As we were doing that I kept thinking, "How is doing this going to help me?" And I just kept thinking, "Stop thinking that and just do it!" [laughter]

Dr. Sears: Yeah. Did you come up with anything?

Laura: No [laughter]. One thing I do is I constantly occupy myself when I'm eating. It used to be TV. I don't watch TV anymore because I just watched too much of it, so I just turn it off. But I'll be looking at Facebook, or have the radio on. I never just sit and eat. I feel like I always have to be somehow occupied while I'm eating. And that actually makes me feel more stressed when I do that.

Dr. Sears: Yeah. And it's a common thing, especially if we're all busy all the time, to think, "What can I get done while I'm eating?" It's a multitasking attitude. And that's fine if you consciously choose to do that sometimes. What you're going to find in this course is that I'm never going to say, "Don't do that, or don't do this." It's just asking, "Did you notice you were doing that, and is this helpful to you, is it what you want to do, and is it going to give you the results you want?" So if you enjoy multitasking at times, that's great. But oftentimes, we're just so distracted that we're missing our experiences in this moment. And we can end up living our whole lives like that. Maybe you're talking to somebody here, but you're really thinking about what you're going to buy when you're at the grocery store, and you miss the chance to really connect with someone. You might begin to discover you're rarely fully engaged with what you're doing in the moment. So this can be a helpful exercise to foster our attention.

Other thoughts about how this exercise can be helpful to us?

Kevin: I'm curious, if you just eat and don't do other stuff, are you bored?

Laura: I don't know the answer to that. That's a good question.

Dr. Sears: For you, Kevin, it sounded like you might feel anxiety if you were to just eat slowly?

Kevin: Sitting down, it would be anxiety, yeah.

Dr. Sears: So in the process of this, we're moving into our experiences so we can develop our ability to pay attention to what's really happening. It's easier to do this with something concrete like a raisin, or our own body sensations, which we'll practice next. Eventually, we're going to work our way to things like emotions and thoughts. And those can be really subtle, but you're already recognizing how our minds are all over the place.

And so, we're going to learn to give that same attention you just gave to that raisin to our other experiences when we choose to do so, whether pleasant or unpleasant. Even for something as simple as looking at a raisin, we can get caught up in thoughts and memories. So it takes some practice. While I'm noticing my thoughts more clearly, I can choose to look at them directly, or I can consciously set them aside for a minute while I go back to what I want to do. With practice, that gets easier.

Of course, the thoughts never completely stop. The goal is not to be blank and feel nothing, like a rock [laughter]. In the East, they call that becoming a "Stone Buddha." The goal is to be a fully alive human being. Your thoughts are going to come and go, but you're less controlled by your thoughts. You have thoughts, but you are more than just your thoughts. So whether you're looking at something as simple as a raisin, or something more complicated like the way you feel about someone, you might notice strong thoughts that won't stop. Rather than struggling with them, you can learn to hold your own thoughts with your attention, and just recognize, "Wow, this is a lot of old crap that just keeps coming back. Maybe I can let that go." Or you might choose to investigate the thoughts, asking, "I wonder if there may be something important in here about a lesson that I need to learn." I can choose to just hold those thoughts with my attention, instead of being driven by them, if that makes any sense.

Some of the stuff I throw out may fall into the category of, "hear me now, believe me later." But the good news is, with practice, you will experience all these things for yourself. None of this is anything you have to memorize or believe in.

Several of you mentioned noticing how all over the place our minds can be. I remember hearing in Sunday school, when I was a kid, that meditation was evil, because if you clear your mind, the devil is going to jump in there. And you know, whatever your belief system, there is definitely some truth to that. As some of you already discovered, if I sit still, if I eat slowly, if I just try to notice what's happening, all kinds of wild, random thoughts arise. Sometimes even bizarre thoughts, right? Just like in dreams, strange things come into your mind. You could attribute that to some external force, but generally, that's just what our minds do. So some people start meditating, but quit because they think it makes their minds worse. But what you'll find is, if you can sit with them, those thoughts will settle down on their own. There's a saying in Zen—don't try to calm the waves on the water by hitting them with a flat iron [laughter]. Instead of struggling with thoughts, we can practice letting them be there, and eventually they will settle down on their own, as your body is settling down underneath. A lot of times, our thoughts are trying to fix the way we're feeling. If we don't like the way we're feeling, our thoughts get busy, busy, busy, busy, which distracts us from any unpleasant feelings in our bodies. As our bodies get calmer, our thoughts will tend to calm down, too. So, we'll be experiencing that too as we go along.

Any more questions or comments on that before we shift to a different exercise?

[Body Scan Exercise]

So, what did you notice during that exercise? What kinds of sensations were present? What was your experience?

Christine: It was hard to sit still.
Dr. Sears: Okay. In what way? Can you describe that?
Christine: I just felt a little uncomfortable and wanted to shift around.
Dr. Sears: Okay. Where in your body did you feel that? Were there thoughts with it?
Christine: Hmmm—there was a tightness in my chest, and I was thinking I needed to be doing something.
Dr. Sears: Okay, so you noticed thoughts, as well as sensations in your chest, along with the discomfort. Anybody else notice an urge to move? Very, very common, especially when you're dealing with stress and anxiety. Actually, when I talked earlier about leaving the room, I

was thinking of a graduate student I had recently in my mindfulness course. She felt like, in the first class, she just literally had to leave the room. She just couldn't sit still for the first couple of exercises. But by the end of the course, well this is going to sound like I'm bragging [laughter], she made a major breakthrough in letting go of her anxiety by learning to just let it be there and allow it to pass on its own. If your own body can't just sit still, and you always struggle with an urge to move, your stress response will be firing constantly. Your parasympathetic system then never has a chance to kick in and let your body relax. It's very normal to feel that urge to move when you're living a busy life, but when you practice coming back to the moment you are in, your body learns to settle down by itself, even in the midst of busyness.

Other things people noticed?

Stephanie: I noticed when we first began, and focused on the left foot, it was amazing how different parts of my body were like, "Well, what's so important about the left foot?" [laughter]. And then we got to the top of it, and you said to let go of it. What I was aware of then was my heart was really beating. From that time on, I was aware of my heart throughout the rest of the meditation. I guess I realized just how strong my heart is.

Dr. Sears: Yeah. Typically, we have no idea what our heart is doing. Or, if you have a lot of stress and anxiety, sometimes you are hyperaware of what your heart is doing all of the time.

Stephanie: Yeah, it's interesting.

Dr. Sears: I'm jumping ahead here, but this is teaching us to stay with what is happening. With anxiety, for example, if I feel my heart beating, it can spark a chain of thoughts. "Is my heart beating too fast? What if something's wrong with my heart? Should I go to the ER? But if I go to the ER, they'll tell me it's just all in my mind, and they'll send me home, and then when it's a real problem they won't listen to me, and then I'll die from a heart attack, and then my family will be without a home, and what are my kids going to do?" I end up worrying about my kids being homeless when all I was doing was feeling my heartbeat. So mindfulness is about noticing, "Oh, I'm thinking a lot right now." I can then decide if it's helpful, or if it's being fueled by anxiety. I can then choose to keep bringing my attention back to the heart, or whatever I'm wanting to stay with, and separate out what my body feels, my emotions, and my thoughts. I will then have more perspectives, allowing me to work more wisely with the anxiety.

Kevin: Stephanie, you could actually feel your heart?

Stephanie: Yeah, I could feel it beating.

Kevin: I don't. I can't feel it.

Dr. Sears: Yeah. I find with time and practice, you can become a lot more aware of your body. I'm actually just on the verge of a cold right now, and I could feel it coming days ago, so I've been trying to rest and take more vitamin C. Unless you do yoga, martial arts, dance, or sports, a lot of us don't notice our bodies until something is wrong, or they're hurting, so we miss important information. Even if you're at the other extreme, where you're hypersensitive, it's important to pay more attention to your body, learning to separate out the thoughts and emotions from the actual sensations that are there.

Stephanie: Well, it was interesting, because I wasn't actually aware of my heartbeat until you said to move all the way up, and then you said let go of the left leg, and then I let go of it. That's when I noticed my heart. And it was like, "Wow!", because I haven't noticed that before. It was a very positive experience.

Dr. Sears: Good. (A few moments of silence.) This a quieter group than I'm used to [laughter], which is fine. Anything else about your experience with the exercise?

Christine: I find it hard to be aware of any part of my body if I'm not moving it.

Dr. Sears: Okay. That is very typical as well. For one thing, physiologically, if there's no motion, it's harder for your brain to sense it. Maybe you've noticed this with a loved one—they put their hand on your lap, and eventually you don't notice it. But when they gently caress, then your brain is sensing the change.

Another piece is that it takes time for your brain to remap itself to be more aware of your own body. Maybe this is a silly example, but I remember watching a science show where they studied a martial artist who had practiced all his moves standing on top of poles. They put some sensors on his feet and they discovered that the bottoms of his feet were much more sensitive than the average person's, because after years of training, his brain remapped itself so that it could be more sensitive. Experienced musicians can feel more in their fingers, or hear more subtle tones, not necessarily because they're born that way, but because the brain will rewire itself through practice. So, the more you pay attention to your body, the more you'll be able to notice things about it.

When things get difficult, it's good to have more information. I remember doing an exercise for a large group of psychologists once, and afterward, someone said sarcastically, "Thanks a lot—I didn't realize my toe was hurting until you told me to notice my body." But the fact of the matter is that it was hurting already. You might choose to ignore it if you've got a chronic pain condition and you're trying to get through a flare-up, but as a long-term strategy, you end up using a lot of energy struggling with yourself if you keep telling yourself not to think about it. If you notice it, you have more options of what to do next, like adjusting your posture, taking an aspirin, or letting the pain be there without adding on more struggle.

Christine: Doesn't your body adjust naturally, if it's a chronic problem, not an acute problem? Like if you stub your toe, and then you break your arm, you're not going to think about your toe anymore, because you have a lot more important things to focus on.

Dr. Sears: Yeah. It's very interesting, because over time, your body typically does adjust. With chronic pain, there are a lot of processes going on. It's very complicated. But we can work with the emotional piece of it. When you're trying actively not to think about it, that kind of keeps it there, just below the surface. Just like with a strong emotion, if I keep fighting it, trying to push it down, telling myself, "I don't want to think about what I've got to do at work tomorrow," it tends to build up. Versus, "Wow, I'm noticing some anxiety about what I don't want to do at work tomorrow," then allowing yourself to feel it. When you open up to it, it will usually get a little worse at first, and then it tends to change, and may even pass once you stop fighting it.

It's a similar process with pain. Telling myself, "I don't want to feel it! I don't want to feel it!" tends to set up a vicious circle of tension and struggle. And I'm not saying this is easy, but instead of tensing up around the pain, I can develop a sense of curiosity about it, and sort of explore it like a scientist. Because, in fact, pain is not a solid thing. It's very dynamic. It waxes and wanes. It gets stronger and softer. It gets sharper and duller. And again, it's not easy, but the more you can let yourself move into it, sort of ride the waves of it, the more it will tend to loosen up and break up a little. We can more directly experience the pain without adding on the resistance that compounds the suffering. This is one of those "hear me now, believe me later" things. It's something you need to experiment with for yourself.

It's the same with unpleasant emotions. We often try to push them away, but if they're already here anyway, we can move into them and explore them. It's just like that raisin. Often we have an idea of what a raisin is, but when you carefully investigate it, you discover all kinds of things that you never noticed. It's actually a very complicated thing. This is even more so for our own thoughts, feelings, and body sensations. We can develop the ability to not just automatically push it away and block it off, but to get in there and ride it out when we choose to do so. So, that's one of the places we're going.

Kevin: I was gratified that I was able to stay through the whole exercise comfortably, because that wouldn't be normal for me probably. And toward the end, my breaths were deeper.

Dr. Sears: Well good. So you were noticing a change in your breath. And that's really important to experience in here, that if you stay with something like stress or anxiety, it can get a little worse, and then it tends to fade naturally. When we struggle to avoid pain or stress that's already present, it tends to get worse. If as we started the exercise, you said, "I don't want to do this!" and ran out of the room, you could unconsciously reinforce a pattern of trying to avoid everything that makes you uncomfortable. And that could lead to a very constricted life.

I think a really good analogy, though it might be overly simplistic, is getting into a cold swimming pool. When you dip your toe in, you might think, "Oh my gosh, it's cold!" And then you keep pulling it out, and dipping it back in, and pulling it back out. Now you feel even colder because your foot is wet and exposed to the air and the wind. If you just jump in, it's a lot worse in the beginning, but if you stay in the water and wait, then your body just gets used to it. You can jump in all at once, or go in slowly, but you have to stay in the water to let the cold feeling rise and pass away.

It's the same with feelings like stress and anxiety. If I stay with it, it feels worse at first, but if I relax into it, so to speak, it just naturally comes down. If I keep jumping out of it, by avoiding it or distracting myself with lots of thinking, I get stuck in a cycle that keeps it going. This is going to be an ongoing theme of this course.

Here's the handout for this week. The first page summarizes the theme of this class, which is automatic pilot, our tendency to often engage in automatic behaviors. So we're going to start practicing paying more attention and asking, "Does this pattern help me? Is it working for me? Or could I do something a little differently?"

The next page is the definition of mindfulness I talked about last week. The following page gives a patient report, which is basically given for inspiration. It's inevitable that some challenges will come up as you begin practicing mindfulness, so you can read about someone else's experiences and challenges in practicing the body scan.

Here are the CDs for you to practice with. All the recordings that you'll need for the entire eight weeks are on there. And depending on your technical savvy, you can save it to your phone, music player, or computer so you can play it anywhere.

I've also listed a few websites where you can download other mindfulness recordings. You'll also find great CDs in *The Mindful Way Workbook* (Teasdale, Williams, & Segal, 2014) and *The Mindful Way Through Depression* (Williams, Teasdale, Segal, & Kabat-Zinn, 2007), which are great books that cover the content of this course in more depth if you'd like something to read between classes.

So the first part of the home practice is to do the body scan once a day until we meet again. The purpose is to develop these "mental muscles," practicing staying with sensations, letting them rise and fall, shifting your attention when you want to, noticing the thoughts and feelings that arise, and coming back to what you want to stay with. As best you can, try not to judge yourself the whole time, like, "Oh, I'm not doing this well—this is a bad day—this is awful." You might even notice, "Oh, I'm having a thought that this is awful, but I'm going to just do the practice anyway." Try to do it with an open-minded, "Let's just see what happens" sense of exploration. That's more of a mindfulness-consistent attitude.

The second part of the home practice is to use the attached sheet to keep track of the exercises you do, so you can check off when you've done them, and you can write comments on how they went. It can be interesting to look back over this and look for patterns, such as how often and how soon you might have fallen asleep. This is only for you—you don't have to turn it in to me or show it to anybody else.

The third thing is to choose one routine activity in your life and practice doing it with more awareness. For example, sometimes we finish a shower so quickly as we're thinking about work that we don't even remember if we shampooed or not. Instead, you can just take your time and pay more attention to what you are doing. You can notice the feeling in your hand as you turn the water on, the temperature change on your body and the smell of the water as it starts to flow, the sparkles on the water as it falls and runs down the drain, all the sensations of washing, and so forth. There's really a lot going on that we don't usually notice. So pick an activity like that once a day as a starting point for bringing this more into your daily life.

Kim: Do we do the same activity every day or a different one?

Dr. Sears: That's up to you. It can be interesting to do the same one the entire week to make it easier to remember, and to notice if the experience of it changes over time, but you can choose a different one each day if you want to.

For the next assignment, anytime you're eating, and you happen to remember, you might choose to pay more attention, as we did with the raisin. And lastly, between now and next week, eat just one entire meal, not painfully slowly necessarily, but just turning off the TV and mindfully paying attention to what you are eating.

I apologize, we've gone over a few minutes. Any more questions?

Laura: I won't be here next week. Do you have the handout for next week?

Dr. Sears: Yeah. Let me give that to you, and we can talk about it after class. If you have any questions you can call or email me.

Any more questions? Okay. See you next week!

6 Session 2

Living in Our Heads

In the original MBCT protocol, this session was called "Dealing With Barriers," because when processing how the week went, participants inevitably bring up a number of challenges they faced, which are very common when beginning mindfulness practice. The protocol manual lists a number of these common obstacles, along with suggestions for processing them with the group (Segal, Williams, & Teasdale, 2013).

The new title, "Living in Our Heads," reflects the broader emphasis of this session, which is about noticing the differences between thinking and direct awareness of experiences and about how often we are captured by automatic patterns of reacting. This is highlighted through more practice with the body scan and with mindful breathing.

This session also introduces cognitive therapy principles through the ABC model and the Pleasant Events Calendar. As therapists, we can sometimes forget how these concepts can be new and very useful for participants.

Throughout the course, we are modeling that dealing with difficult situations begins with noticing things as they are. This is why each group begins with a mindfulness exercise before talking about how the week went. However, I do allow for any burning questions or comments so that participants are not distracted with trying to remember something during the exercise.

Session 2 Transcript

Dr. Sears: Well, let's get started, unless there are questions. I prefer to process how the week went after we do the initial exercise, to start off with this moment, unless there's anything you just have to get off your mind to be able to concentrate on the exercise. Okay, good.

[Body Scan Exercise]

Kevin: A half hour ago, that would have been impossible.
Dr. Sears: Mmm-hmm. That was 22 minutes long. It's impressive to be able to sit still that long after only a week of practice. It's good to let your body settle down. Sounds like it was pleasant for you?
Kevin: Mmm-hmm. This has been one of my hardest days in a long time, in terms of anxiety and depressive symptoms, getting

Dr. Sears: Okay.

Kevin: So, I'm grateful that I'm so calm all of a sudden. I can't believe this. I've been bouncing off the walls most of the day.

Dr. Sears: So to stay with this exercise, did you notice, even as we sat down, that the feelings were there? And then what happened—did they kind of dissolve, did they get worse at first? What was your experience during the exercise?

Kevin: They got better, calmer, almost immediately when I sat down.

Dr. Sears: Okay. Good. What did others notice?

Christine: I found myself getting very fidgety, though not here as much as at home. I don't know if it's because I have other things I feel like I need to be doing, but I find myself looking at my CD player, how much time is left. I don't know why I can't get my nervous system calm enough to just relax into the moment.

Dr. Sears: That's very, very common. I think one of the benefits of having the structure of a group like this is that it helps you stick with it long enough to get past that point. I still remember someone coming up to me and saying, "I'm going to get up at 5 a.m. every day and meditate for an hour." Maybe he was feeling inspired, or maybe he thought he was going to impress me or something, but I told him I didn't think that was a good idea. After a couple of days, you realize that 5 a.m. is way too early, and an hour is such a long time, so you just give up. Having others practicing with you helps you understand what's normal and what you can do to make it a better experience.

So for you, discovering that you feel more agitated, you might tell yourself, "I feel worse! Why would I do this? It's not fun! I'm going to quit!" With all of us going through this together, there is some support and guidance. So how was it today? Did you notice it changing?

Christine: Well at home it gets worse, well, I don't know. The longer the time goes on, I still feel that way. Here, I don't so much. But whenever I'm at home I have trouble keeping my mind on what I'm doing, and I want to get it done so I can move on and do something else. I don't know why.

Kevin: Are there other people around when you're doing it?

Dr. Sears: It can often be just a mental habit, continuously asking, "What's next, what's next, what's next?" Even, "Wow, I've got 5 minutes of downtime. I could do this or I could do that." It's a big shift to be able to realize that right now, in this moment, this is all I need to be doing. I can be right here with whatever I'm doing. It takes some time and practice. If you stick with it, you'll pass through the agitation, and your stress response will fire much less often.

Now the good news is, you don't have to give up getting stuff done. Sometimes I'll have people come to me and say, "I'm afraid if I do mindfulness then I'll lose my edge. If I stop or slow down, I'll just kind of collapse, and I won't get anything done. I won't be as productive." And of course I always say, "Well, just try it as an experiment. Don't take my word for it." And inevitably they say, "Wow, I'm actually much more productive now, because I can focus on my work and get it done much more efficiently. I'm not wasting energy thinking of all the things that I can't do while I'm doing what I'm doing."

Any other things about this exercise we just did before we talk about how the week went?

Stephanie: I can stay with it, then all of a sudden I'll realize I've already made a grocery list, or done something else in my head. It's interesting how my mind will slip off, and then I have to just gently pull it back. Just a little delay.

Dr. Sears: Yeah—and that's wonderful. Even if that's all you got out of the entire exercise. You noticed where your mind was, and you gently brought it back. That's that idea of waking up to the moment.

Stephanie: Interesting.

Dr. Sears: As I said during the exercise, our minds will typically beat us up for being gone 80% of the time, but actually being present 20% is great!

Kim: Yeah. That actually helped me. I was like, "Hey! Yeah! All right!"

Kevin: I had that too. That's a ratio that is so generous [laughter]. Where else in life is it okay to just get 20%? [laughter]

Dr. Sears: It's so true! Even during a mindfulness exercise, we can start putting pressure on ourselves. I can start beating myself up. "I need to pay more attention! I'm wandering off!"

Christine: I think it's funny that you use the word "celebrate." I don't usually think of having a party because I'm here 20% of the time.

Kevin: I think it's great. I know. I love that!

Christine: You use that word on the CD.

Kevin: Celebrate coming back to awareness.

Dr. Sears: Yeah—I can't say that I made that up myself. I've heard my teachers use it.

Christine: I never thought about actually celebrating that.

Dr. Sears: Yeah. We get in such a learned habit of "I've got to do this, or I've got to do that." Your brain actually has a tendency to look for the worst. It's a survival mechanism. If I can find the worst, then I can survive longer. It's a mindset shift to look for the positive.

Kevin: If compassion for the self, being good to myself, is one of the cornerstones of mindfulness, then celebrating 80/20 is right in there. Yeah.

Dr. Sears: Right. Noticing what's going well in addition to what's not. Noticing I'm coming back to where I wanted my mind to be. And then you can build on that, instead of only thinking, "Well, I failed 80% of the time. I'm no good at this and I'll never do it right."

Kevin: It feels silly at first, because most of us were expected to get 90 out of 100 in school, and caught flack for it if we didn't. So being able to celebrate 20 out of 100—I like it! It feels good.

Dr. Sears: Yeah. Anything else about this exercise? It's really important to understand that you're not going to always have this wonderful, positive, relaxing experience. If you are already feeling anxious, you can practice letting it be here. If relaxation comes, it's most likely to come from just staying present, from letting go of struggling with yourself. If you work really hard at relaxing, it tends not to happen. It's a paradoxical thing—if your attitude is, "I'm just going to notice whatever's here, and I'm going to just let it be here," then your body often relaxes as sort of a side effect.

Christine: My energy therapist here taught me how to move my energy down to my feet by just thinking about my feet. Before that, I would never just think about my feet. It's kind of an odd thing to do.

Dr. Sears: Yeah. You know, a lot of us, especially somebody like me in academia, often feel like we live in our heads, from which our bodies sort of dangle. One of the goals of this course is to become a more whole and integrated person.

Christine: That's cool.

Dr. Sears: Yeah, so this is one way of practicing. But again, it doesn't mean it's going to be positive. There are going to be days when I check in with my body and I notice, "Wow, I'm in a lot of pain," or "I'm really feeling anxious or stressed right now." That's more information, so I can make better choices. I can choose to go do something to take care of myself, or I can decide to push through and get through this important business meeting first, or I can just stay present with it. It starts with more awareness, instead of pretending it's not there.

Kevin: I had an interesting experience. I was at Serpent Mound a few days ago for World Peace Day. All over the world there were drumming circles and celebrations going on at the same time. A local group met at Serpent Mound, and a good majority of the people stayed overnight. I tried to, but it got cold, surprisingly cold. There was actually frost. I thought, "Wow, look at this sky! I haven't seen this many stars in months! I'm going to open the sunroof on my car, and it's going to be perfect. I'm going to do the body scan, and it's going to be beautiful." And you know what, by the time I got into my car to do that, that energy had

	already shifted, and I didn't want to do it then. And just being there among all those stars was already a scan.
Dr. Sears:	Yeah. You were already present in the moment. That's great.
Kevin:	I was already present in the moment. Yeah. And then I slept for two hours, and woke up with popsicle toes. I drove home at like 2:00 in the morning. It was too cold! [laughter]
Dr. Sears:	That reminds me of an important point—we're going to be doing a variety of exercises over the course of these eight weeks. Some people tell me, "Oh, I love the body scan, and it really helps me." Other people say, "No, it's not for me," and they like some other exercise better. It's all meant to foster more awareness. So if you can, keep that open-minded experimentation attitude going.

We already started talking about it, but how did the week go in general with the home practice? |
Kim:	I fought with you a lot.
Dr. Sears:	Fought with me? Okay. Good. That means you were taking it seriously and testing it out, checking it out.
Kim:	I just kept thinking, "Why can't I think about my shopping list right now? What's so wrong about that? Why can't I do this and that? Why do I have to keep coming back to this? Why can't I worry if the dog needs walking right now?"
Dr. Sears:	Well, you know, the answer is obviously that you can, but are you choosing to do so, or is it a compulsive, "I can't help myself"?
Kim:	Oh, I'm sure it's compulsive. But it was easier to blame you [laughter]. To be mad at you.
Dr. Sears:	Right. Exactly. I'll take the fall [laughter]. You bring up another good point, though, because you can also go to the other extreme. There's a famous Zen teacher who said, "When eating, just eat. When walking, just walk," meaning to just be present in what you are doing. One day a student came in, and the teacher was reading the newspaper as he was eating his breakfast. The student said, "Teacher! You've always told us when eating, just to eat, yet here you are reading the newspaper while you're eating!"
Stephanie:	Oh, that is hilarious!
Kevin:	I know what he's going to report.
Dr. Sears:	The teacher said, "When eating and reading the newspaper, just eat and read the newspaper." The point is that you don't want to go to some kind of extreme of trying to always be completely present.
Kevin:	I heard that story about Chogyam Trungpa.
Dr. Sears:	I had heard it about Seung Sahn.
Kevin:	They tell the same stories [laughter].
Dr. Sears:	Yeah, I'm not surprised. It's about not getting stuck in the extremes. So if my mind goes off a lot, I just notice that.
Kim:	And then I'm like, "I'm really talented that I can do all this at once! Isn't this really cool? Wait—I'm stressed!"

Kevin:	But, can I ask you something? When you were doing that, like doing a list in your mind, and walking the dog, do you think that you were kinda getting things done? Getting things planned when you were thinking about those chores? Or do you think that if you would have stayed with the body scan, that those chores wouldn't have gotten done?
Kim:	I don't think I even went that far. I think it was just unintentional thoughts coming to my mind. And it wasn't so much I felt like I had to do it or it wouldn't get done. I mean, I was able to suppress it, and you know, put it to the side. And then, it was like, it kept happening. I can recall this has gone on as long as I can remember. My son does it, and he has ADD, because he can't stay on one thing. But he's just the way that I am, where in my head, I'm on to the next thing, and on to the next thing. And did I do that last thing, and did I complete it?
Dr. Sears:	And your brain can't always tell the difference between a thought and a real threat, so it tends to react to each of those thoughts with a tiny squirt of stress chemicals.
Kim:	And it's great, because as I'm becoming more aware, and able to slow it down, and bring myself back, I think it's also something I can work with my son on.
Dr. Sears:	Yeah, you can model it. Another important thing is the attitude we take. I know you were using a shortcut in saying the word "suppress," but you'll find that the more you try to stop this kind of thinking, usually the worse it gets. We're practicing to foster a kind attitude toward ourselves, like, "Oh, thank you, mind, for trying to help me right now by making that list, I appreciate that, but right now I'm going to come back over here." Because the worst thing we can do is get in a battle with ourselves, and spend a lot of time and energy on that. Kevin brought up a good point about how we think all this thinking is so helpful and new, and how important it is, and that we better not forget it. But usually when we start to look at it, it's just the same old stuff over and over again. Peter Matthiessen said he went to his Zen teacher and asked, "I'm a writer, and sometimes I have all these creative thoughts while I'm meditating. Should I always practice just letting them go?" The teacher suggested that he keep a pad of paper next to him, that way if a brilliant, creative thought comes in, he can just write it down and then let it go.
Kim:	That's great!
Dr. Sears:	So, if you know you could write something down, suddenly the pressure's off.
Stephanie:	I keep a notebook by my bed, so I don't sit there trying to go to sleep, and I write it down, and then that's it.

Dr. Sears: Exactly, yeah. Now, we'll talk more about thoughts in future sessions, but writing them down is another way of stepping back from them, rather than getting lost in them. Once you get perspective on them, you can relate to them differently, or do something with them more consciously. I know someone who teaches mindfulness to actors and artists to help them become more creative. Once the habitual mind chatter settles down, you'll make room for and recognize more original and creative thoughts. It's interesting.

Anything else about how the week is going? It takes some effort to establish a regular mindfulness practice, which is why this session is called "Dealing With Barriers." It can be challenging to just find the time to do it, to keep up the motivation, and to work with resistance when it comes up. For many people, the only time they ever sit still is when it's time to go to sleep, so that is fairly common, so just noticing that too.

Kevin: I'd like to share something not so easy. I think I got a lot of practice with mindfulness—a lot. Because, my anxiety at this point is serious enough that I'm not working, plus the fact that I only relocated here a couple of months ago from overseas, so I haven't been looking for work anyway. So, I don't have a lot of things to distract me during the day. So, I'm looking at mindfulness, and looking at the quality of my thoughts a lot—not hiding from it—definitely not hiding from it. But, it's hard. Really hard.

Dr. Sears: Yeah. So maybe you could consider this a training period to get yourself in a better place, and then when an opportunity comes along, you'll be better prepared.

Kevin: A work opportunity? Right.

Dr. Sears: Yeah. So, even if for some reason you find that you're not doing the mindfulness exercises, you can make that an opportunity to practice. What's the feeling that comes up when I start hesitating about doing it? Can I feel the resistance in my body? What thoughts are coming up? By checking into my experience, I'm already practicing mindfulness.

Stephanie: It took me a couple of days to get the CD down on my iPod. So, the first night, and then the next morning, I tried to do my own little body scan, and I did it a whole lot faster than the way you did it. But that was helpful. And I had a friend come in. I actually left the class last Monday and went to the airport to pick her up. But I wanted to share with you, it was funny, I shared with her the experience I had with the raisin, and how just being with the raisin and putting all my focus into this room, how I was just really aware of all the sadness I'd been carrying, and how I cried. And she said, "Wow, just imagine what would have happened if you had stared at a prune!" [laughter]. That's what friends are for!

	We laughed and laughed. We actually went to Niagara Falls. We left on Thursday, and she and I just had a ladies' getaway, and . . .
Kevin:	*Thelma & Louise!*
Stephanie:	. . . to be able to be there, and I used all the five senses. The mist—at one point I was tasting the mist! Even though I give myself maybe a 20% on my homework, I was able to be in the present moment at different times, and to be there was good. That was a gift.
Dr. Sears:	And that's the point—just to practice what you want to be able to do more consciously. It is up to you how you want to do that. The formal exercises are important to give us a solid foundation, but the whole point is to enrich our daily lives.
Stephanie:	And I was thinking, as you were talking about barriers, part of me was a little hesitant to listen to the body scan, because part of me was afraid to have to look at that sadness again.
Dr. Sears:	Right, sure.
Stephanie:	And I'm going to have to look at that sadness. I know that if I don't look at that sadness, it could end up as depression, or issues that I'll have to deal with later.
Dr. Sears:	Yeah. Interestingly, I could literally pull the manual for this course out and show everyone a list of all the common barriers that come up. Strong emotions are very common. We're all so accustomed to being busy, busy, busy, busy, and now we're learning to be more present. Old stuff will just bubble up sometimes. It may often be nothing, just popping up out of nowhere and disappearing again. Other times, like for you, it's much more immediate and raw, because it's so fresh for you. But we can say, "Okay, it's here." We may not need to do anything with it. We don't have to automatically fight it, or hold it in, or spend a lot of energy struggling with it. Here it is, I may or may not choose to engage with it in this moment, and it will inevitably change.
Stephanie:	And going through a divorce, I know that the more that I'm able to be present right now, the less that I'm going to have to deal with the residue later.
Dr. Sears:	Right. And recognizing that, this isn't the scientific term, but that it's just going to suck for a while.
Stephanie:	It is! I know!
Dr. Sears:	And not to sit here and pretend, "Oh, I'm going to feel good about my divorce." No, it's an awful thing to go through! But here it is, and I'm just going to feel it. I'm not going to add another layer of awful on top of what I'm already feeling. Just working with what's already here.
Kevin:	Can I share something that happened today about mindfulness? I was at my doctor's office. I didn't have an appointment, but I needed to pick up a product. And I was having one of the worst

mornings I've had in a long time, so I needed to just take a little walk before I got out of my car to go in there. So I saw sort of a side street, off the back of the office, and I started exploring back there. Someone had set up a real nice armchair under a real nice pine tree in the woods, behind the building. So I was kind of just back there checking it out. But then a guy came out of the building for his break from work, and he said, "What are you doing back there?" And I said, "I'm a patient of this doctor's practice." I was a little snippy, actually, sort of like, "You don't need to know." And he said, "Well, there's been some thefts back here, so I was just checking things out." So what started out as a snippy little confrontational thing quickly changed. He could probably see that I was in some distress, so he kind of shifted, and he said, "What are you seeing him for?" And I was just going to blow him off at first, but then I said, "Well, I'm dealing with some anxiety issues." And he said. "Aw, man, I know exactly what you're going through. I had that for a while a couple years ago." And it ended up being a really good interaction. And I think that was partially from being mindful of how I was feeling. I didn't hide, and he was able to see me and see what was going on. And later in that walk, I was in a little patch of the woods, and I saw a butterfly, with black and white wings. I just watched it, for like 10 minutes.

Dr. Sears: It's amazing how often we'll just pass by things like that and not even notice. It's interesting to also notice changes in the way we relate to people. Inevitably, over the course of these eight weeks, people will tell me, "You know, my partner seems a lot nicer since I started this group." They often get along a lot better with their partners, even if the partner is not practicing mindfulness. What seems to be happening is, they notice things like, "Wow, I was snippety just then," and so they stop, or apologize, and then the partner is more relaxed and is not snippety back at them, and then they feel closer. It's interesting.

Christine: I think mindfulness just brings about a feeling of gratefulness for what you have.

Dr. Sears: I certainly have found that.

Christine: My nieces and nephews that live here in town—I spend a lot of time with them, and they just make me laugh. I have lots of fun running around with them. I saw them this past week, and I can realize that it's great that I have them, that they cheer me up and make me laugh. So I think the mindfulness helps them as well to be a little bit more appreciative of what they have.

Dr. Sears: I think so. Kids are just much more naturally aware, and just have that curiosity and that wonder in everything they see. I think we often get that beaten out of us as we get older, and . . .

Christine: We can end up just telling kids what they need to do, and how they're not behaving or whatever, instead of being grateful for the opportunity to spend time with them.

Dr. Sears: Yeah. All right, before talking about one of the themes for today, I want to start off with a scenario. This is only a couple of sentences long. See if you can imagine the scenario, and imagine what you would be thinking and feeling if this happened to you. So you're walking down the street, and on the other side of the street, you see somebody you know. You smile and wave. The person just doesn't seem to notice, and walks by (Segal, Williams, & Teasdale, 2013).

Maybe you've had that experience, or you can imagine it. You're just walking down the street, and all of a sudden, there's somebody you know. You wave, and they just keep walking. So, what kind of thoughts or feelings would pop up for you? There's no right or wrong answer to this—just throw some out.

Christine: Did they see you?

Dr. Sears: Yeah, just wondering first of all, did they even see you?

Kevin: One possibility is feeling slighted.

Dr. Sears: Uh-huh. Yeah.

Kevin: Another possibility is thinking, "Oh, they probably didn't see me. They're probably concentrating on something else. They probably had something else going on."

Dr. Sears: Right. Yeah. I might think they didn't like me, or I did something wrong. I might wonder if they're okay, if they had something else going on, if they were concentrating on something else.

Stephanie: You wonder if that was really them.

Dr. Sears: Yeah, "Was that really who I thought it was?" And then you kind of do the thing where you act like you raised your hand to brush it through your hair [laughter].

Kim: I think I might be really embarrassed, wondering, "Hey, did anybody see me?"

Dr. Sears: Embarrassed, yeah.

Christine: And then you do that thing where you recognize the face, but you can't remember their name, or where you know them from, and so you avoid talking to them because you can't remember their name.

Dr. Sears: Yeah, right. Good. All these different things. It's interesting, because there are lots of possible reactions. Sometimes people say, "Oh, they hate me, they heard about what I did at the office, and they're not going to talk to me anymore." People have a lot of different interpretations, but of course the point is, it's a totally neutral situation. We have no idea. Right? It could be anything. It could even be that they left their glasses at home, or like you said, they're concentrating, or . . .

Stephanie:	Or maybe they're having a bad day, too.
Dr. Sears:	Maybe they're having a bad day, and don't want to speak to anyone.
Kevin:	The point is, it may have nothing to do with us.
Dr. Sears:	Right, right.
Stephanie:	That's funny.
Dr. Sears:	But our minds fill it in.
Stephanie:	But then I would also wonder what people think that I waved and they didn't wave back [laughter].
Kim:	Yeah, that's what I thought about the embarrassment. "Oh boy, people are going to wonder why."
Dr. Sears:	Right. So, one of the themes that we're going to talk about is how situations, thoughts or beliefs, and our feelings interact with each other. If I have the *thought*, "Boy, people are going to think that I'm stupid!", then I'm probably going to *feel* embarrassed, or if I *think*, "They really hate me," then I'm going to *feel* a little more depressed.
Kim:	Interesting.
Dr. Sears:	And the opposite too, right? If I'm already feeling really depressed, I'm more likely to think, "Here's one more person that won't even listen to me. Nobody likes me!" Or if I'm in a great mood, and they didn't notice me, I'm more likely to think, "Oh, what a loss, because they would have had a great time talking to me today" [laughter]. Thoughts and emotions influence each other.

Let's draw this up on the board. It's called the ABC Model. "A" stands for "activating event." The technical term is "antecedent," or the thing that happens first, or before. "B" is "belief," or could be "behavior." "C" is "consequence," what happens afterwards, which could be a feeling in this case. So, basically something happens, and then I have a thought or belief about what happened, and then a consequence follows—how I'm feeling about it, or what I'm deciding to do about it.

I was just listening to a lecture by Robert Sapolsky (2010). He's a stress researcher, and has a great understanding of the physical stress response, but he jokingly talks about how thoughts mess up the research. We have a sophisticated series of chemical reactions, but if you believe that the event is not stressful, then none of it happens. Your appraisal of the situation, or how you interpret the event, completely changes your reaction to the event.

In a really dramatic way, Stephen Covey (1989) tells a story of being on a subway train and trying to get some work done. There's a father there with two or three kids, and the kids are just jumping all over the place, yelling and kicking and bumping into people. Stephen gets increasingly frustrated, because the dad is just kind of staring at the floor. Finally, he goes up to the dad and says, "Can you please control your children—I'm trying to get some work done here." The dad looks up and says, "Oh, uh, I'm really sorry. I just found out that their mother got killed in a car accident this morning." Of course, Stephen immediately feels bad for them, and offers to help with the kids. The belief about what's going on totally shifts how you experience the situation.

Now, I'm not saying you should just believe happy thoughts, like, "Oh, this person is being abusive to me, but I really think at heart they're a nice person." I'm not talking about creating a different belief to change something that's really bad in reality. What's important is to first stop and notice our own thinking, and see how it fits with the situation.

When I was a doctoral student, I did anger management groups at the Veteran's Hospital. That was an interesting experience. They often missed the "B." One of the veterans told me about an activating event of a guy calling him a name, so of course he hit the guy. Almost as if the guy just came right up and grabbed the veteran's fists and pulled them into his own face. My task was to help them realize that there is a tiny belief or thought in there, in between the name calling and the fist hitting the face. For them, it might be, "If I don't show them physical force, I may not feel like a man," or "I feel like I'm less than other people, so I need to get physical to show I'm strong," or some other thought, or some feeling underneath the anger, like fear or loneliness.

Stephanie: I have to protect myself—that's interesting.

Dr. Sears: I'm not going to test this out, but I would hope that if someone came in and called one of you a name, you'd think, "What's going on with this person? Obviously, they have no idea what a wonderful person I am. How sad that they have to resort to name calling to relate to people. How unfortunate that they will miss out on the opportunity be my friend" [laughter]. We would have a belief that, "Wow, if I hit this person I would go to jail, why would I want to do that?" Maybe we would leave, or call the police, or do something to fix the situation.

Kevin: Depends on what kind of mood I'm in.

Dr. Sears: Right, and that's important. If I recognize, "Wow, I'm not in a good mood," then that's going to mean that I better pay attention to my choices, and try not to put myself in a situation where I could act out.

Kevin: More likely to lead to a scene.

Dr. Sears: Yeah. What I would tell these guys is, "Wow, it's amazing that you allow a complete stranger to rule your life like that, because they could put you in jail just by calling you a name. That's giving somebody a lot of power over you." Now it's much easier to see this in other people, right? But to see that in ourselves—what are the automatic thoughts that we have, and the automatic beliefs we have, that get us in trouble sometimes? Maybe we get caught up in a belief that kept us safe in the past, but now it gets us in trouble.

So, a big part of this course is going to be about paying more attention. What are those thoughts? So far you're starting to notice things like grocery lists, which are fairly benign, but eventually we'll start to notice more and more subtle beliefs and thoughts that affect the way we respond to difficulties. One of the goals is to have more awareness, so we can consciously choose the best way to move forward. We may even realize that we don't have to say or do anything, and unpleasant feelings may just pass on their own. Or maybe we notice this does require some action, but we can do it in a way that doesn't make us suddenly look like we're the ones who are angry and out of control.

Have you ever been in that situation? Somebody says something to you that's just so mean that you get very upset, and then you say something harsh, and now suddenly you look like a mean person. And they're like, "Oh, see, I don't know why you're out of control like this." And then it's like, "No, you were the one who made me like this!" [laughter] We can automatically get pulled into that kind of a situation. We can learn to pause and notice, "Wow, I'm having a strong reaction right now. What's the best way to handle this?" I may certainly have a right and a need to express my anger, or to set some boundaries, but it's important to do it consciously, and avoid reacting in a way that gets me in trouble.

Stephanie: And so, we become aware, and we notice the belief, and then we can—we consciously choose to change the belief?
Dr. Sears: That gets a lot deeper, to try and change the belief.
Kim: A consequence doesn't have to be negative.
Stephanie: No, but our belief will affect our action, and that will change the consequences, right?
Dr. Sears: Well, you're trying to create a little bit more . . .
Stephanie: I want the answers [laughter]!
Dr. Sears: The answers will come with time. The goal right now is to . . .
Christine: Just notice it.
Kim: Be aware, breathe in.
Dr. Sears: Right. Just notice it. Expand a little bit of a gap, and then choose what you're going to do about it, if anything, instead of automatically . . .
Stephanie: So "C" could be "choose" instead of "consequence"?
Dr. Sears: It could. Absolutely. It's a lot like the 24-hour rule with email. You get this really infuriating email, and you get an urge to write a scathing reply, and then you hit send, and then you can't take it back.
Christine: Wait 24 hours before you send it.

Dr. Sears: Right. The rule is ideally to wait 24 hours.

Kevin: But don't forget to reply.

Dr. Sears: It's about taking some time and making sure you are saying what you really want to say, instead of something you might regret later, and looking like you're out of control.

Stephanie: Or if you don't reply, they may get more out of control [laughter].

Dr. Sears: Yeah. There are a lot of variables that our thinking can come up with. We start by expanding that gap.

Stephanie: That's good.

Dr. Sears: So with these veterans, instead of just hitting right away, taking a few seconds to ask, "If I hit, what would that do? Is that the end result I want to get from this situation? Are there other ways to get what I want out of this situation?" Again, expanding the gap between "A" and "C." And longer term for them, of course, is to examine the belief that "I'm only a man if I hit people." I can begin to discover other ways that I can show that I'm a man, or other ways to feel strong. When other areas of my life start to get better and more fulfilling, I have less of a need to prove to other people how good I am. All these different things start to come out. So, ultimately, you could start to change and question, but in that moment, you're just trying to notice it, and then ask yourself, "Is this really the way I want to act in this moment? Is there something I can challenge about this belief right now? Is this truly what I believe?"

Stephanie: That's good.

Dr. Sears: So, we're going to have you practice noticing thoughts, feelings, and behaviors. I'm going to pass around these handouts. On the very back, you'll see the "pleasant events calendar." Interestingly, Kevin has already demonstrated exactly what I'm talking about, which is being able to notice some small positive event. I've noticed this group is a little more positive than most. I've had people in some groups say, "I just can't seem to find a positive thing in my day."

Stephanie: Aaaww.

Dr. Sears: And again, that's because we're so used to noticing what's wrong. It requires a little bit of a shift. So we'll do this to practice noticing, and to practice breaking these apart. Breaking apart the components of our experiences like this gives us more leverage to work with them. So instead of, "Here's this awful thing, and I don't know what to do with it," I can break it down into "Here's what my body is feeling, here's what my thoughts are, here's what my emotion is, here's the action I can do." When you start to break it down a little bit, you can intervene at any one of those levels instead of just getting overwhelmed.

So, remember one positive event per day, and then break it down. Here's the example in the handout (Segal, Williams, & Teasdale, 2013, p. 175). "Heading home at the end of my shift.

Stopping, hearing a bird sing." That's interesting, because Kevin saw a butterfly in his case. "How did your body feel, in detail, during this experience?" Again, trying to break this down a little bit. "Lightness across the face, aware of shoulders dropping, uplift of corners of mouth," a smile. "What moods and feelings accompanied this event?" "Relief, pleasure." "What thoughts went through your mind?", "that's good, how lovely." Just noticing, what thoughts and feelings are there? And in the last column, if you're writing this down at the end of the day, "What thoughts are entering your mind now, as you write this down?" "Such a small thing, but I'm glad I noticed it." Now this is important—you don't have to make it positive. It's possible that even as you're experiencing it, you're thinking, "Yeah, the bird's lovely, but I hope it doesn't poop on my house." Whatever it is, just write it down without judging it and thinking that you have to try to make it all positive. Right now the goal is just to be more aware. You might write down, "This is dumb, I hate this homework assignment" [laughter]. Whatever it is.

Kim: "I'm mad at you again" [laughter].

Dr. Sears: "Again! When is this ever going to end?" [laughter] But the point is to start to break open our experiences. Here's the thought. Here's the feeling. Here's the body sensation. Those are the three areas we can start to break apart. And then, later on, as you can probably guess, the next assignment is going to be practicing with unpleasant events. It's easier, I think, to start with something positive and break it down, and then you can do the same thing when you get stressed out, when something negative is happening. Because then I can intervene at any one of those levels. Instead of thinking the whole thing is overwhelming, I can notice and work with my body sensations, my thoughts, or my feelings.

Stephanie: Interesting.

Dr. Sears: Breaking those apart. So does that make sense as the home practice assignment? You're obviously welcome to do it all day long if you want to, but just write down one per day to practice with.

Christine: Are we supposed to do the body scan again? Every day?

Dr. Sears: Yeah. There's one more exercise I want to do first, and then we'll go over the home practices. But yeah, that'll be another piece.

I was just thinking about one of my meditation teachers, Stephen K. Hayes, who had us do an exercise in which we were asked to remember something pleasant that had happened that day. At first, I had trouble remembering positive things, because my day had been very busy, and I had rushed through traffic to get there. What really surprised me was once my brain got into that mindset, I could remember hundreds of pleasant things. Very often, we don't notice things that are going the way they're supposed to—we notice when they go wrong. Once you get in that mindset of noticing things to be appreciative about—not in a forced way, but just recognizing them—the more your mind gets in that habit, and the more positive things you notice. And we have studies showing that people who write down even a few things they are grateful for on a regular basis are happier.

Stephanie: Interesting.

Dr. Sears: Any other thoughts or questions so far before we do a different exercise?

[Exercise—mindfulness of breath]

Dr. Sears: So, how was that exercise? What did you notice? That was just a few minutes long since we're almost out of time.

Kevin: I was 80% right on the breath.

Dr. Sears: Wonderful.

Kevin: That's surprising.

Stephanie: I was just digesting part of what you said before, instead of just being right here. It was amazing how I was like . . .

Dr. Sears: Oh, okay, yeah, because I just loaded your mind right before with a bunch of things to think about.

Stephanie: Because even though I was here, I was just processing that. It was just interesting.

Dr. Sears: That's such a great attitude. "It was interesting." That's exactly what we want to develop. Not, "I'm fighting my brain," just noticing that what my brain does. And I think that's important, because we don't want to have a blank mind. Just noticing, "Oh, this is what my mind does," and then bringing your mind to where you want it to be.

Anything else on that? Okay, that'll be another one of the assignments to practice at home. It's such a simple thing—just watching your breath—but our minds often go all over the place. You can imagine how much our minds want to jump around if we are facing something unpleasant, or something complicated. This is practice for consciously choosing to stay with something. The breath is one of those interesting things that is both conscious and subconscious. Especially when you have asthma or anxiety, sometimes when you're told to look at the breath. . .

Kim: I didn't want to bring it up, but this is hard for me, because I have asthma. I think this is hard for me, because when you're on the nebulizer, you see your breath, and you're panicking, and when I think of the breath it doesn't give me peaceful, soothing, relaxing feelings.

Dr. Sears: Right. And that's really important. So there's a faith piece—not that you have to have blind faith, but just enough to try it out. Initially, watching your breath will make you feel more anxiety, but the more you stay with it, and the more you practice, the more quickly it will change and even pass away. As you know, the anticipation and anxiety that something could happen causes you to change the way you breathe, like feeling a need to protect your breath, so you breathe a little more shallowly. But shallow breathing is more likely to trigger anxiety and the stress response, which makes it more likely that you'll lose your breath and have another attack. So practicing staying with our experiences helps break the vicious cycle our thoughts and emotions get us caught in.

Kim: Yeah, change my belief.
Dr. Sears: Well, yeah, through experience.
Kevin: "Mad at him."
Kim: "I'm going to be mad at him again" [laughter].
Dr. Sears: "Still mad. Still can't breathe any better" [laughter].
Kim: "Monday mad."
Dr. Sears: All right, let's look at the handouts and the home practice. As I mentioned, today's theme was dealing with barriers. So, just recognizing these challenges are normal, staying with them, and riding them through. We're doing the body scan again this week, so the next page has a few more tips and some inspirational things to consider as you continue that practice.

And then, funny as it might sound, three whole pages about breathing. The first couple are instructions for the practice, and things to consider as you're doing it. One of the points on the next page is that the breath can be sort of a barometer of how you're feeling. When I first started working with people with pretty serious anxiety, I really remember being struck by how quickly and shallowly many of them were breathing and didn't know it. They just thought breathing that way was normal. I would tell them that if I were to breathe quickly that way from my chest, I would start to have tingling in my fingertips, feel light-headed, and my heart would race. It's just a physiological response. People found it very helpful just to learn to breathe more deeply from the diaphragm, even though it might feel like they were suffocating a little at first. Sometimes breathing alone really changes the way the body feels, and how often you're having panic attacks. But anyway, just getting more in touch with and noticing your breath can have quite an impact all by itself, in addition to practicing paying attention to things as they're happening.

So again, keep doing the body scan for this coming week. And at different times, do the mindful breathing practice. Now, if the only time you have is at the end of the day and you need to do these two back to back, that's okay, but ideally you want to focus on doing each one separately. You can set a timer for 10 to 15 minutes, and just practice feeling your breath, noticing when your mind wanders, and gently bringing it back. You can also listen to a recording if you want a voice every now and then just to say, "Remember to follow your breath."

The third thing, as we talked about already, is the pleasant events calendar. Once a day, just noticing and writing down the details of a pleasant event that happened.

And the fourth thing is just to pick some new daily activity to do with more awareness. Now some of you may have already been doing a different activity every day, and that's okay. If you were doing the same one all last week, pick a different one this week. Again, the idea is to practice bringing this into your daily life, instead of only when you're doing an exercise, or only when you're in class. So just pick some other activity in your daily life that you want to pay more attention to.

And that's it. Any other questions, comments, or thoughts? All right, thanks, everybody, for staying with it. Like Woody Allen said, 90% is just showing up. It's especially true for mindfulness.

Stephanie: That's great. Thanks, Richard.
Kim: I apologize for being late.
Dr. Sears: No problem. Anytime you're late, just slip into the room and join right in.

7 Session 3

Gathering the Scattered Mind

In the original MBCT protocol, this session was called "Mindfulness of the Breath," but the new title makes more explicit that we can notice how scattered the mind tends to be and that we can use the breath or the body as an anchor for bringing awareness back to the present. This session introduces a number of new exercises to demonstrate how mindful awareness can be fostered through a variety of activities.

An important part of this session is introducing the idea of staying present with intense physical sensations rather than automatically avoiding them or struggling with them. This will evolve with time but can begin with simply choosing to notice when a painful sensation or an itch is present during a mindfulness exercise. Participants may shift their bodies or scratch if they choose, but they can also begin to look at the changing nature of the sensations, perhaps using the breath as an anchor if they cannot stay with it. In this session, you might highlight noticing and choicefulness, and in later sessions, you can invite them to move into and stay present with difficulties. During inquiry, you can ask how this way of relating to difficult sensations is different from how they might normally do so and how this way may be useful.

These concepts are also emphasized in the Unpleasant Events Calendar, in which participants are asked to notice one unpleasant event each day and pay attention to the associated thoughts, feelings, and sensations that arise.

One of the other ways mindfulness helps is by filling the limited capacity of the brain's attentional channels with present-moment experiences, making it difficult for ruminative thoughts to take hold (Segal, Williams, & Teasdale, 2013; Teasdale, Segal, & Williams, 1995). If I am filling my awareness with the various sensations of breathing, there is less room for negative thoughts. However, this should not be confused with avoidance. If I am breathing to escape my unpleasant feelings, they will tend to get worse. This difference can be subtle, but it is very important. For this reason, I tend to first emphasize experimentation with staying present and moving into experiences to counter habitual avoidance patterns.

This session illustrates the importance of flexibility. For instance, in inquiring about the in-class exercise, the participants kept shifting to the topic of pain. While in most cases I would simply redirect to present-moment experiences, this topic was very important to the participants and illustrated some crucial points, so I stayed with the digression before coming back to the curriculum. If clients don't "buy in" to the practical value of mindfulness practice, they are at risk of dropping out of the class. Just as we teach participants in the class, we can model moving into a difficulty that is pulling for our attention, explore it, and then return our attention to where we need it to be.

Of note, one of the participants, Kim, decided to drop out of the class the week before. She emailed to say she had some life circumstances come up, so I told her she could begin again with the next round of groups. Perhaps she could not get past her "mad."

Session 3 Transcript

[Talk before class about acupuncture]

Stephanie: He can show us how to be more mindful during painful experiences [laughter].

Dr. Sears: All right, let's get started. Actually, this is the most intense day as far as new exercises go. Actually, they're not intense in the sense of needles poking your body, but just a lot more new ones, so we should go ahead and get started, unless there are any burning questions or comments to get off your mind.

So remember, all of this is in the spirit of experimenting and noticing what's going on with your mind and your body as we do these. We'll start with a sitting meditation.

[Exercise—mindfulness of breath, body, staying with unpleasant sensations, sounds]

Dr. Sears: So what did you notice during that exercise? We did several different things.

Kevin: You hit the nail on the head for me—it's lower back pain.

Dr. Sears: Okay—I saw you sort of moving in your seat a little bit.

Stephanie: And I don't know if it's sympathy pains, but my back kind of bothered me a little bit afterwards. I think it was the way that I was sitting. And I don't have back pain. So. . .

Laura: Same here! I usually don't have any back pain, until you asked us to notice if there was any! [laughter]

Stephanie: Isn't that funny?

Kevin: It's weird, because I think I'm in pretty good shape, but I think one thing is that I lug this big bag around, and it's too heavy. I think that might be the problem.

Christine: How is it helpful to focus on pain?

Dr. Sears: How is it helpful?

Christine: Yeah—because it seems to make it a little worse.

Dr. Sears: Yeah. I think this is a really good point, and let me just hit pause on that question and come back to it in just a moment. Because

	I was thinking it is possible that my suggestion had something to do with it, but more likely . . .
Stephanie:	Get those needles out [laughter].
Dr. Sears:	But more likely, there was probably a little tension there anyway.
Stephanie:	Exactly.
Dr. Sears:	Maybe it wasn't enough to be like, "Oh my gosh, my back is killing me!" It was like, "Oh, now that I'm looking, maybe there is a little something there."
Stephanie:	It was awareness.
Dr. Sears:	And so what can happen is, if you don't check in every once in a while with your body, tension can build up. It goes up your back, and then your shoulders get tight, and then your neck gets tight, and then you start having a headache. By noticing, you might then decide to carry that bag differently before it creates a problem. I remember I started having back pain years ago, and someone just asked me a simple question, "Do you wear your wallet in your back pocket?" It turned out that sitting on my wallet created a small shift so that my back had to strain a little bit on one side. Once I started wearing my wallet in my front pocket, the pain went away.
Stephanie:	Interesting.
Dr. Sears:	So first of all, noticing it's there gives us information. Sometimes somebody will tell me, "Yeah, I was feeling fine until you told me to notice my body, and now I notice my toe is really hurting!" But it was already hurting anyway. Now that you know it is hurting, you can try to ignore it again, or loosen your shoe, or stretch your toe, or take some aspirin. But, before I answer Christine's question, what did you notice when I said go ahead and stay with it and notice . . .
Kevin:	I did that. I did as you suggested, and I kind of just stayed with it and tried to notice more specifics about it. And I did notice subtleties and shades from inside it. It wasn't really constant.
Dr. Sears:	Right.
Kevin:	Little, tiny oases of nonpain in the overall pain experience. And then maybe a little bit sharper.
Dr. Sears:	Right. Well good. I don't know how much time that was, but it was very brief, and my concern is if I do it too briefly, you don't have enough time to notice how pain tends to change. The initial experience is usually exactly as you said—it gets worse. "Oh, I forgot that my back was hurting, and now that I'm noticing it, it feels worse." But if you stay with it long enough, you'll start to notice subtle things about it. But it doesn't mean that it melts away and now you feel great.
Kevin:	Nope.
Dr. Sears:	Yeah. But it starts to change a little bit. It's one thing to hear it, but it's important to experience for yourself how it's not constant and unchanging. Pain is not a solid "thing," like you can knock it

out, or like it's all or nothing. It's kind of alive and changing. You described it very well. Those gaps start to open up—moments when the pain isn't quite there. It waxes and wanes. Sometimes it's sharp, sometimes it's dull.

The attitude we take toward pain can be very important. Fostering curiosity and exploration, like, "Wow, what is this?", even though it's not easy, or pleasant, right? If I resist and push back, then I'm fighting and struggling with myself. After all, it's my own pain, it's my own body, and yet I can set myself up to struggle and fight.

Even physiologically, what can happen is, if my knee is hurting, then I start to tense my muscles around it, because my body subconsciously wants to protect my knee so it doesn't get hurt again. And I might even start leaning more weight on the other leg so I can take pressure off of the hurt knee. But then my spine becomes misaligned, and my shoulders and neck need to compensate, and I can unwittingly make my entire body hurt much more.

So, first developing a more conscious awareness of what I'm doing. Do I want to do this? Is it helping? Does it make it worse? Especially tensing muscles around a painful area—the strain often increases the pain, but it becomes a habit when you've had chronic pain for a long time. So, that's another one of those "hear me now and believe me later" kind of things. You really just have to experiment with it.

Also, this is one more approach. I'm not suggesting that every single time you feel pain, you must drop everything you're doing and really feel it. But if every time pain comes up, your automatic habit is to pretend it's not there, or just watch TV, or distract yourself so you don't have to feel it, in the long term it can become worse. Obviously there are times when you know the pain is temporary, like when you're getting a cavity filled at the dentist, or you're having a flare-up, and you may just choose to distract yourself to get through it as best you can. But if it's a lingering kind of pain, it's a bad habit to just always try to pretend it's not there. By moving into it, you really start to change your relationship to it.

As always, if people are having trouble with this, or it's getting worse, or if more people are having pain and want to talk about it, we can spend more time on that in future sessions.

What else about the exercise we did today? Breathing, and feeling the entire body, and sounds, and we had the distractions going on outside the room.

Christine: With the pain, when I do the body scan, I notice pain that I didn't realize was there.

Dr. Sears: Okay.

Christine: I can even feel where I had surgery on my left leg. And there's a scar there. That part's not painful, but I can feel a sense of something different there. If I do have pain in other places, it puts a focus on that. I had planned to ask you about that today anyway. Is that a good thing?

Dr. Sears: Okay—while we're on the topic of pain, let's talk about that. So, obviously when there's a painful part, it's going to pull your attention. Are you able to keep shifting back along with the CD? . . .

Christine: Shifting back?

Dr. Sears: To whatever part the CD is saying to focus on? Do you notice you're stuck on the painful parts?

Christine: Well, I just notice that the pain gets worse, usually when I focus on it. I just didn't know . . .

Dr. Sears: Yeah, it does. So what happens next? Are you able to stay with that? When it starts to get worse, what happens?

Christine: I just try to do whatever you're saying to do, and I move on, and just try not to think about it quite as much when we move on to the next area.

Dr. Sears: Okay. We're moving away from the body scan next week. But, as difficult as it might sound, just see if you can keep that open mind toward what you're noticing, "Oh, isn't that interesting, it's getting worse now that I'm looking at it." Fostering that curiosity toward it, and just observing.

There's actually a CD set called *Mindfulness Meditation for Pain Relief*, done by Jon Kabat-Zinn (2010). There are two CDs, one talking about the concepts, and one with mindfulness exercises. So that might be helpful. Staying with the pain, even for a few minutes, sounds a little counterintuitive when you're thinking, "I don't really want to feel the pain." And again, you'll notice right away that it gets worse when you pay attention to it, but eventually it starts to break up, and the intensity changes. And once you have that experience, that you can just move into it and it breaks up, it changes your attitude toward it. Because initially, you think, "Oh, it's getting worse now! I *really* don't want to think about it!" So, you go back to trying not to think about it. And while you're trying not to think about it, you're really thinking about trying not to think about it [laughter]. So yeah, it takes a little bit of faith, but what's the alternative? It's there. It's already in your body. Ignoring it is helpful sometimes, but it takes a lot of energy to keep doing that. So, we can sometimes choose to stay with it and relate to it in a different way.

Anything else with the exercise we just did today?

Laura: The sound—when you were talking about listening to sounds. With my hearing loss, I have just a little bit of ringing in my ears. I don't notice it most of the time. I really noticed it.

Dr. Sears: Oh, okay. Interesting.
Laura: It's kind of, almost annoying.
Dr. Sears: So you noticed the sound, and then you noticed annoyance arising. And how quickly our brain wants to label a sound, or immediately think about it. And so it's an interesting phenomenon—if I'm busy thinking about the sounds, it's like the thinking is another layer, and I'm not going to hear the actual sounds as well, if that makes any sense. It's like, if I'm talking all the time, I'm never going to hear what somebody else has to say. So if I'm talking to myself all the time, which is what thinking is, I'm not going to hear what's going on around me. The thoughts are an extra layer. Now, obviously, sometimes it's a wonderful thing to think about what's going on, but when it's a compulsive habit, then it can get in the way of the actual experience. It's almost like looking through this dirty window at something. When you clean the window, things are so much more clear and vivid.
Kevin: I can hear a high-pitched sound that sounds like insects or crickets.
Dr. Sears: Yeah, up in the ventilation. Yeah.
Kevin: And it reminds me of one of the alarms I use on my cell phone to remind me of certain things. I use the cricket sound effect.
Dr. Sears: Oh, okay. So you noticed the thought, "Oh, that's my phone ring." Yeah. That can be interesting to notice. People often comment on the clock. "Yeah, I didn't notice the clock until it was quiet, and then I noticed it, then I couldn't stop, then I realized I wasn't hearing it anymore."
Christine: I can't sleep in rooms that have battery-operated clocks.
Laura: Yeah, I can't stand it. I have to put it away in another room or something.
Dr. Sears: Like a water torture kind of thing . . .
Kevin: I have a clock like that. I have to put it in the drawer and close the drawer.
Dr. Sears: So again, it's all about just noticing where we're at right now. Once you become aware, you're then in a better place to decide what you want to do about it, if something needs to be done, like putting the clock in the drawer. But it starts with, "What am I noticing? What is happening, and how am I reacting to it? Am I getting into any old patterns? Is it helpful? Is it not helpful?" So we just start with noticing. In that exercise, we shifted to a different sense, of sound, instead of feeling the body. Eventually we'll shift to looking directly at our own thoughts.
  Good. Anything else on that exercise?
Stephanie: I like when you said imagine your whole body breathing. I had a couple of breaths there where it was like, "I got that!"
Dr. Sears: Oh good!

Stephanie: Then it was like, "Wow, that was really cool." Then I kind of lost it. I was trying to get it back. So, it was kind of funny. Because it felt really . . . it was like two or three breaths. Then I think I tried to control it or something, because I kind of lost it.

Kevin: Two or three—that's already a lot. Here, that's really advanced.

Dr. Sears: Yeah, well, I was going to say, even to have that experience, that's good. And then you noticed that a thought came up, and you noticed your experience changed.

Stephanie: It was cool.

Dr. Sears: Yeah. Well good. What did others experience when I asked you to feel your entire body all at once?

Laura: I had a hard time just staying still during that. Just fidgeting. I get uncomfortable very easily or something.

Dr. Sears: Yeah, and that's actually very common as well. Did you notice where the restlessness comes from? Do you feel it in any particular place in your body?

Laura: No. Just a need to move.

Dr. Sears: Okay. Have you noticed now, this is already the third session, is it getting easier or worse when you do the exercises?

Laura: Oh, actually a little easier.

Dr. Sears: Okay. That's my experience too. Over the course of the weeks, your body learns that there's a time when being ready is helpful, and there's a time when just being still is regenerative, so it's nice to have more options.

So, how did the previous week go in terms of the home practice, including the pleasant events calendar?

Laura: Oh, I forgot to do that!

Christine: I think to focus on the positive always helps me, to think about things and to appreciate the good things that have happened every day.

Dr. Sears: Okay, so it was a positive experience for you?

Christine: Yeah, as opposed to focusing on, "Well this went wrong, and this went wrong," to try and pick something positive out, even the small things.

Dr. Sears: Well good. Anything else about the . . .

Kevin: I think probably if we learn how to appreciate a whole bunch of little, small things, I can see that having a cumulative effect.

Dr. Sears: Yeah.

Kevin: I'm not there yet, but I could imagine it [laughter].

Dr. Sears: I wish I could remember the details, but there was an experiment where people who were asked to write down even a few things they were grateful for on a regular basis became happier.

Laura: I have a Facebook friend who at the end of every day posts three things that she's grateful for that happened or that she experienced that day.

Dr. Sears: Ahh, that's great!

Laura: Yeah, it's pretty cool. I thought, "I need to start doing that."

Dr. Sears: Yeah—and it's fascinating to me that research confirms that. And it doesn't mean that you have to stretch it or make things up like, "Well, all my hair didn't fall out today, I'm grateful for that!" [laughter]. But just the habit of looking and noticing what you do have really does make a difference.

Laura: And her things can be very simple, like some kind of food that tasted fantastic, or some little thing. And it's really cool to read them. Even though it's not my life, it's still cool, like "Oh, that's great that you're expressing this positive thing!"

Dr. Sears: Yeah—that's a good point.

Kevin: Well that's good that you have that reaction to it, rather than "Who cares?" [laughter]

Laura: Well I think it's because she's stating that she's grateful. But, yeah, sometimes people post stuff, and you're like, "Well I don't care." But just because she's expressing gratitude, it makes it more pleasant to read. More interesting.

Dr. Sears: Yeah. And in a very literal sense, you're sort of rewiring your brain to appreciate that, and allowing yourself to feel more happy and appreciative. Our brains often automatically look for what's wrong, and often ignore what's going well. And when your whole life becomes, "Let's always look for what's wrong," that creates a stress response that really takes a toll on your body.

All right, anything else about the previous week before we do another exercise?

Laura: The only time I did the pleasant experience thing, I was on vacation all week, so I just forgot all about it.

Dr. Sears: Well, you were living it! [laughter]

Laura: I was on a road trip with my sister, and we were driving from one town to the next, and there was this beautiful sunset, and I was like, "We gotta pull off so I can take a picture of this!" Then I thought, "No, just enjoy it." And I thought about the homework we were supposed to be doing. And yeah, just experience it, and don't feel like you have to get a picture of it.

Kevin: Yeah. Capture it! [laughter]

Dr. Sears: That's a really interesting phenomenon, and I've thought about it myself, and I've heard other people talk about that too. It's like the camera puts another layer between me and the experience. When you're back, it's great to have the pictures, although nowadays, with digital pictures, I've got thousands that I don't have enough lifetime left to even look at. But yeah, just to be fully present with what's going on rather than thinking about how you're going to capture it the whole time.

All right, the next exercise is called the three-minute breathing space.

[Exercise—3-minute breathing space]

Dr. Sears:	That might have been a little longer than three minutes, but that's the idea of the three parts. What did you notice during that exercise?
Kevin:	I got really good deep breaths.
Dr. Sears:	Mmm-hmm. Okay.
Kevin:	And the minute we were focusing on the breathing, I naturally found myself taking a regular-length inhale, and then sort of a pursed mouth, really slow exhale, and it felt really good.
Dr. Sears:	Well good, that's nice. It's almost like you felt what your body needed in that moment?
Kevin:	Yeah. I didn't want the exercise to end! [laughter]
Dr. Sears:	Good! What else?
Christine:	You said to focus on your thoughts, and I found myself thinking, "Okay, how am I going to explain what I just experienced?" Like putting it into words already.
Dr. Sears:	Yeah.
Christine:	Which wasn't helpful.
Dr. Sears:	You are already hitting on a very subtle thing we'll get to in the next few weeks. We tend to define who we are by our thinking, but we can begin to recognize we are more than just our thinking. I have to use words to express myself, but there's a lot more to who I am.

Another common thing is not finding any thoughts when you first start to look for them. It's like, "Well, where are my thoughts? I thought I had some! But wait, that might be a thought, that I don't have any thoughts going on right now!" It's because we're so used to being in our thoughts, it's hard to notice what our thoughts are. Thoughts can become so habitual that we don't even know we think certain ways about certain things. So, just noticing our thoughts is a good start for shifting how we react to things. As we talked about last week, your thoughts and your feelings interact with each other. If I have certain kinds of thoughts, it's going to make me feel a certain way, and if I'm in a certain kind mood, I'm more likely to have certain kinds of thoughts. So I can start to recognize that when I'm having a lot of negative thoughts, I must be in a bad mood. That's a very mature thing to do, rather than automatically taking it out on other people. It means, "Oh, I need to take care of myself right now because I'm having a lot of negative thoughts."

Anything else about that exercise? We're going to be practicing that one during the week coming up. |
Laura:	When you asked us to notice our emotions, and then to look at our thoughts, I felt happy, and yet I was also feeling stressed about work, thinking about that. How can I be stressed and happy at the same time?
Dr. Sears:	Yeah. Anybody else notice something like that?
Stephanie:	I noticed I was tired. Mentally and physically.

Dr. Sears: Yeah, I think it's possible to have dozens of feelings at the same time. But we tend to just not notice, or we notice the strongest one, and eventually start to find that there are all these different layers. With practice, you might come to more often recognize, "Wow, I'm holding on to this thing from work. I wonder what that's about?" And it may not be about anything in particular, so you just start to sit with it. Maybe it goes away, or maybe it gets stronger. But you can start to tease all that out, instead of carrying it around all the time.

Kevin: I think on a lot of levels in our lives, it's supposed to be A *or* B. Democrat *or* Republican. A thousand other examples. Why does it have to be A *or* B? That's oversimplified.

Dr. Sears: Sure.

Kevin: Isn't it a little bit of A, a little bit of B, a little bit of X . . .

Dr. Sears: That fits with my experience.

Stephanie: A little bit of F [laughter].

Kevin: Yeah—all of the above!

Dr. Sears: Yeah. It's a common expression to say "I have mixed feelings" about a person or a job, but we often don't really notice much about those feelings. They're sort of running in the background, and have an effect on how we're feeling or what we're thinking. So we're just going to expand what we're noticing, which gives us more options for what to do with it, if anything.

All right, good. Anything else on that exercise before we shift to the next one?

Christine: If our thoughts are about all the things we need to do, I mean, weren't we supposed to not be thinking about those things?

Dr. Sears: Well, what you're going to find, and there's actually research on this, the more you try not to think, the stronger your thoughts tend to get.

Kevin: Yeah—I believe it!

Dr. Sears: In a technique called "thought stopping," I just tell myself, "Stop it!" if I start thinking something I don't want to think. But the research shows that usually just makes it worse (Wegner, Schneider, Carter, & White, 1987). The more you try to not try to think about it, the more the thoughts come. Because now you're feeling more stress, and your thinking is your way not to feel stress. You're trying to think it out, and you stress yourself by trying to stop your thinking. In Zen, they would say that's like trying to smooth out waves with a flat iron, which just makes them worse. It's good to start with noticing, "Oh, wow, the water is really wavy right now."

Christine: Oh, boy!

Dr. Sears: So your thoughts are all over the place right now, but eventually you'll notice they will settle. Another analogy is to imagine a cup of dirty water. Instead of shaking it all up, if you just let it be still, the dirt will start to settle down to the bottom, and the water gets really clear. Same with meditation. Eventually the thoughts start to settle down, and there's a sense of clarity there. But not always—the goal is not to have no thoughts, it's just to recognize, "Wow, this is what my mind does." And I notice my mind keeps going over there, but I want my attention to stay here. So the thoughts may even still be present, but you just bring your attention back to where you want it to be.

And that's the discipline part. My thoughts go off, I bring my attention back. My thoughts go off, I bring my attention back. They may even keep going off just that quickly, but eventually you can stay with what you want to stay with longer and longer.

Kevin: What's that thing they say? Okay, don't visualize a pink elephant right now.

Dr. Sears: Right. Wasn't that an East Indian idea, that if you think of a monkey when you take medicine, it won't work? Which of course shows the paradox of how you're not in control of your own thoughts.

Okay, the next thing we are going to do is mindful stretching.

[Exercise—mindful stretching—slow neck rolls, and lifting each hand toward the ceiling and holding it there for a few minutes]

Dr. Sears: What did people notice? How was that exercise?

Laura: My arm felt sooo heavy when we were going back down. Did anybody else feel that?

Christine: My hands got really cold, because I could feel the blood coming from my arm to my fingertips.

Kevin: That's good awareness.

Christine: It felt numb for a while.

Kevin: I noticed as my right arm got above the halfway point, I started to feel a little bit of back pain. And on both sides, I felt the giving of the fabric of my shirt.

Dr. Sears: Nice. Again, it's just about noticing all the changing. Even subtle things like clothing. If you've ever had clothing or a shoe rub you raw, you may not notice it until the end of the day, when there's a giant blister. And again, I'm not saying that we need to always be hyperaware, like, "Oh, I feel a sensation behind my left thigh right now" [laughter]. But just by noticing more, we'll have more options. This is also teaching us another way to relate to difficulties. When things get stressful, we can start to approach it by noticing our bodies, rather than compulsively analyzing it with our thinking. Of course, especially with an external problem, thinking can help, certainly. But when it becomes our only habit, it can get us into trouble sometimes. We're going to learn to reexperience things more often with our bodies.

The other piece is, this exercise is done in motion. It's not just sitting still and waiting for things to change. We can practice being more present as we're moving and interacting with people. Again, I think people who do yoga, martial arts, or dance often figure this out on their own.

Stephanie: It's kind of a form of meditation.

Dr. Sears: Yeah, absolutely.

Stephanie: Because you're moving so slow you're more focused on it.

Dr. Sears: Yeah. And eventually, even if it's normal or fast speed, you can certainly still be mindful. I think it's easier to slow it down for practice.

Anybody else experience that sensation of, "I kind of want to put my arm down, but I'm going to hold it here anyway?"

Stephanie: I was glad when you said time to bring it down [laughter].

Christine: What was the point in keeping it there longer than what's comfortable?

Dr. Sears: What would you guess? What might that help you to learn?

Kevin: I think similar to what Richard just said, about when you find yourself in some kind of uncomfortable situation, instead of instinctively shrinking or shying away from it, or running for cover, whether physical or mental, to stay with it a little bit longer, and try and maybe learn something about it before you run.

Dr. Sears: Very well said. Yeah. Now this was very, very short, probably less than 10 minutes long. I've been in groups where they'll make this 45 minutes long, just the stretching part.

Stephanie: Wow.

Dr. Sears: And of course yoga routines can be an hour or more. So the idea is, noticing how I may automatically want to just pull away when I feel uncomfortable. Which is always an option, though we're already pretty good at that, right? [laughter]

Stephanie: Well, you also gave us the out that if we're in pain we could stop.

Dr. Sears: Yeah, if you needed to, sure. Let me ask you, Christine, what did you experience when you decided to keep it there? You could have taken it down at any time, but you decided to go along, for whatever reason. What was that like? Did you notice it became worse? Was it just uncomfortable the whole time? Or did you notice some changing things?

Christine: Probably a little worse, I think. I have trouble with my right shoulder, and I could hang in there like you said and see what happens. I think that made it a little worse, but I wasn't in so much pain I felt like I had to bring it down.

Dr. Sears: Okay, so, a couple of things. One is, maybe that specific exercise, with a bad shoulder, may not be so good to do. The other thing is, even though that might have seemed like a long time for some of us, it might not have been long enough. There just comes that point when your thoughts tell you that you've got to put it down, but if you just stay with it, your resistance begins to ease up, and you find maybe you can hang out there a little longer. Your brain often resists more when you're not the one in control of the situation. Your brain fights it, with, "I hope it's over soon! I hope it's over soon! I hope it's over soon!" Then finally, you escape the discomfort. We can learn to let go of the struggle, with, "Here I am, and this is the way it is right now." You kind of breathe into it, and stay with it. "I don't like this. I'd like to put my arm down, but this is the way it is right now, and I'm just going to stay with it for a little bit." And there comes this moment when you almost forget that you're waiting, and you relate differently to the sensations.

So, as you just mentioned, this is not only about physical discomfort, this is a model for emotional discomfort. "I don't like this. I'm stressed. I'm worried about it. Well, it's here anyway, so I'm just going to stay with it." It often gets a little worse when you decide to just feel it. But instead of always struggling to avoid it, you recognize you can also choose just to stay here and move into it, and then that's when it may even pass by itself.

Stephanie: I also noticed that when we first started, I had tension in my shoulders.

Dr. Sears: Oh, okay.

Stephanie: And as we've been talking, I just noticed, "Aw, yeah, I don't have tension in my shoulders anymore." I thought that was interesting.

Dr. Sears: Well, good. In this program, we put more emphasis on learning principles of cognitive therapy and psychology, but the original program, called mindfulness-based stress reduction, has a whole lot of yoga. Almost every class has maybe 45 minutes of it.

Stephanie: Wow!

Dr. Sears: That's about all the yoga we're going to be doing, as a class. Now as homework, you're encouraged to do more, if you're in a class already, or if you already have or would like to start your own routine.

Stephanie: Mmmm. Interesting.

Dr. Sears: Just practicing yoga by itself is stress reducing, even without adding other mindfulness exercises, because it is a way of being active and present. But another thing that often comes up, especially with chronic pain, is you stop using your body that much, because you're afraid of hurting yourself, and you become inactive. So, carefully done, very carefully done, yoga can help stretch your muscles back out, and tone and heal some of the other muscles that were tightened by stress and by a subconscious effort protect the painful areas. Yoga helps with chronic pain because it's getting your body moving again, loosens up the muscles, and teaches us to stay present with the sensations.

So, in here, we're using stretching as another vehicle to get at this mindfulness sense of just staying present. Whether it's pleasant or not, just staying present with it. You'll become aware of more choices, and will notice the discomfort changes, and sometimes even passes. If you find yoga helpful, you can join a class or practice with a video. And if not, then you can do other exercises. It's just one more way of getting in touch with our experiences.

Anything else before we shift to the last exercise?

All right, so for the last one, we're going to stand up again. I'm going to throw out a few instructions and then just let you go. Everybody here knows how to walk, because I've seen you do it [laughter].

[Mindful walking exercise]

Dr. Sears: All right, so what did you notice during that exercise?
Christine: My ankles cracking. I don't know if anybody else could hear them.
Dr. Sears: Okay, yeah.
Stephanie: I noticed that as I was walking, it was easier for me to go off somewhere in my mind, to start thinking about something else. It was like, "Well, I don't think I'm supposed to be doing that [laughter]—come back!"
Dr. Sears: Okay. That's interesting. Anybody have the opposite, where because they were moving, and especially moving slower, that . . .
Kevin: I was very focused on the steps.
Dr. Sears: So you were very present.
Stephanie: Isn't that interesting.
Dr. Sears: That's another reason why we try different exercises. People respond differently.
Stephanie: I walk every day. I have a big hill in my neighborhood. And that's kind of my "all right, time to start processing stuff" time. I think I kind of went there automatically.
Christine: It gets your blood flowing while you're walking, too, so that's probably part of why you think more clearly while you're walking.
Stephanie: That's interesting.
Dr. Sears: Looking at the brain, there's actually a process where once you learn to do something like walking, it's stored subconsciously in an area called the basal ganglia, so you literally don't have to think about it. You know, when babies learn, everything is new, and they're trying to figure it out. That's why it can be good when you're learning to pay attention again, to go slowly. Anybody notice you almost forgot how to walk when we slowed it down?
Laura: Yeah, it's really hard to walk that slowly.
Dr. Sears: Yeah, you have to pay more attention, because we don't walk slowly very often. At a normal speed, it's easier to slip into automatic pilot. And like you said, it's not a bad thing, but if we have a habit of always thinking when we walk, we might automatically go there. You could also choose to walk at a normal speed and decide you're going to just look at the trees, or just feel your body as you're walking. It's not that one's better, or right or wrong. The

	question is, can you choose which one you want to do, instead of always doing it automatically?
Kevin:	I noticed at the very beginning, each step was very ponderous and tense, and then I kind of turned a switch after about 30 seconds, and realized, "Wait a minute, I can step much lighter, and it's okay. I won't fall down."
Dr. Sears:	Wonderful. Again, this theme I want to keep highlighting is to notice that when we start something, we often have lots of ideas about what is going to happen. But if we stay with our experiences, and separate out our thoughts, what we were afraid was going to be so awful may just break up a little bit and change.
Laura:	When we started, I just felt really silly.
Dr. Sears:	It was an odd thing to be asked to do.
Laura:	I then thought, "Don't feel silly. Just try to experience it and see what happens."
Dr. Sears:	Yeah.
Laura:	I was thinking, "If anybody sees us, we're going to look ridiculous!"
Dr. Sears:	Right—somebody opens the door, and we're all walking around like zombies [laughter].
Laura:	So it was hard to get that thought out of my head so I could just experience it.
Dr. Sears:	Yeah. And that was very short, because we're running out of time for today, but ideally we would have more time to stay with it, and typically, the strange or silly feelings will pass. Consider all the ways that this happens in our lives. You're going to ask the boss for a promotion, and your mind goes everywhere, and you feel a little uncomfortable, so you back away from it. Versus deciding that something is important enough to do even if it does make you uncomfortable. Of course, feelings are important messengers, so you may decide it is not a good time to ask for a raise, or that something really does need to be avoided, or that the feelings are just baggage from long ago. I can pay attention and make it more of a conscious choice. "I'm noticing this reaction, but that's normal. Let me just wait and see what happens."
	Backing away from something that makes you anxious usually makes you feel better right away, but if my habit is always to avoid things that make me uncomfortable, my life can become very limited. Now in here, there's some peer pressure, so if you had strong thoughts of, "This is silly—I'm sitting down," you might feel even sillier sitting down, because everyone else is still doing it.
Stephanie:	They may be looking at you [laughter].
Dr. Sears:	But in general, if you're by yourself and you're about to do something, and decide, "No, I feel silly, I'm just not going to not do it," you've reinforced backing away from things you don't like. Now of course we all do this, but if it becomes my only option, it can

get me in trouble. In the extreme, I can end up with something like agoraphobia, because if I always back away from everything, at some point the anxiety may get so bad I don't even leave my own house to avoid feeling anxious.

That's obviously an extreme, but the idea is, if it's important to you, you might choose to stay with uncomfortable feelings longer than you might normally have thought to, and then it gets better. Remember the analogy of the cold swimming pool. If you just stand on the edge of the pool, dipping your foot in and out, you will never get past the discomfort. There's that initial, "Holy cow, it's so cold!" But when you get into the water, whether slowly or by diving in, you feel colder initially, but if you stay in it, your body adjusts, and it feels great, and you enjoy yourself in the water.

This is probably stretching the analogy a little, but I was working with someone with anxiety who would do things that made him anxious, but struggle the whole time, and then get out of it quickly, and of course he didn't feel better. It was like he was jumping in the pool and running to the other side to get out really fast. You have to stay in the water and not fight it constantly. You have to let go of the resistance and wait it out. It's hard to stay with unpleasant experiences—we just want to jump out of there immediately. But staying present gives us more choices.

This practice also helps us stay present for pleasant experiences, right? Laura mentioned seeing a sunset. How many times have we barely noticed something pleasant like that? "Yeah, it's a sunset, but I have to think about what I'm going to cook for dinner," or you're always jumping into something else in your mind. It's just nice to have the ability to choose more often to stay with an experience.

And again, I don't want to go to the other extreme where we feel like we "have to" be in all our experiences all the time, like giving ourselves another thing we have to do [laughter]. It's just about developing more flexibility, so we're not as stuck in things.

Kevin: That walking exercise made me think of a beautiful little book. I'm not sure how to pronounce his name correctly—by the Vietnamese/French . . .

Dr. Sears: Thich Nhat Hanh?

Kevin: Yeah. Thich Nhat Hanh. *Peace in Every Step.* A beautiful little book. And it's about walking meditation.

Laura: And that's the title, *Peace in Every Step*?

Kevin: Yeah.

Dr. Sears: He's written a lot about mindfulness from a Vietnamese Zen perspective. It's good stuff.

All right, anything else on that exercise?

Here are the handouts for today. The first page talks about the underlying theme, mindfulness of the breath. We did a lot of different exercises today, but breath has been important in all of them, as a way of gathering our normally scattered minds. You can read through this later. The next page is about the three-minute breathing space. There is a track on the CD to guide you through it, but here are the written instructions with the three steps.

So, for the home practice, the first item is to do the sitting meditation we did at the beginning of class every other day for the next week.

The second thing is, on the alternate days, to practice some kind of physical activity in a mindful way. Does that make sense? So one day you'll do sitting, and the next day you'll do something physical. The activity is up to you. If you do yoga, by all means, you can do your yoga routine. It could just be stretching—if you remember stretches from your high school gym class, that's fine too. If you're really into basketball, you could practice feeling all your muscles as you're shooting the ball, pay attention to what you see, hear, and smell, and practice noticing when you get lost in your thinking. You know, really it could be any physical activity for that matter. For instance, there's a Zen archery practice, using massive bows, where you meditate on drawing the string with your whole body, feel the release, and watch the arrow fly. So, as it describes here, the whole point is to have a more direct way to connect with your body and the awareness of what's going on in the moment, because the body is the place where emotions often get expressed. A lot of times, we don't even know how we're feeling until we can tune in. And when overwhelming thoughts come up, we can practice experiencing them from a different place, like the body. The last part just says if you do have any physical health issues, obviously use good judgment in what's appropriate for you.

The third thing is to practice the three-minute breathing space three times a day. The suggestion is to decide in advance when you're going to do that, so you don't have to keep trying to decide when to do it. In the coming weeks, you'll be practicing it anytime during the day you start to feel stressed or overwhelmed. A funny thing can happen if you only do it when you're stressed—your brain might start to associate it with stress. So, basically what I want you to do is practice the form of doing it, so when you need it you already have the skill of becoming more present with things in just three minutes.

Christine: That's the one that's on the CD?
Dr. Sears: Yeah, and the written description is in the handout. So that's up to you—you can listen to the CD, or put it on your phone, or the instructions are pretty simple if want to do it from memory.

And the last part of the home practice is to record an event like we did last week, but with unpleasant events.

Stephanie: That would have been a good exercise last week for me.

Dr. Sears: So let's look at the example (Segal, Williams, & Teasdale, 2013, p. 211). "What was the experience?" "Waiting for the cable company to come out and fix the line, realizing I'm missing an important meeting at work." "How did your body feel, in detail?" Again, starting to break it down. "Temples throbbing, tightness in my neck and shoulders, pacing back and forth." "What moods and feelings accompanied this event?" "Angry, helpless." "What thoughts accompanied this event?" "Is this what they mean by service? They don't have to be responsible, they have a monopoly. This is one meeting I didn't want to miss." So, just whatever it is. Again, this is just for you—you don't have to turn this in. Just write down whatever it is—you're practicing noticing what thoughts come up when you get stressed or upset. And then, lastly, "What thoughts are on your mind now as you write this down?" Maybe it's the end of the day, and you're remembering the event. What thoughts are popping up now? They could be negative or positive—just write them down. Don't feel like you have to change them or give the event a silver lining, like, "I learned patience from that experience." It could well be, "That was awful! I hope I never have to go through that again!" Because right now, we're just practicing recognizing and breaking apart our experiences. This is a thought. This is a feeling. This is a body sensation. We often get those all mixed up, so we're practicing investigating more closely. We can then deal with our difficulties from any one of those three angles instead of just feeling overwhelmed by it all.

Any questions or comments on that?

Christine: What's the last sentence on that assignment about—"What are the unpleasant events that 'pull you off center' or 'get you down?'" (Segal, Williams, & Teasdale, 2013, p. 209).

Dr. Sears: That's a bigger question to look at, starting to recognize, "What are the little things that start to pull me off center, or start to get me down?" This is especially important for preventing longer-term issues, like falling into a depressive relapse, or having panic attacks, or getting overwhelmed with stress. We can practice noticing the little things in our day that start to pull us off balance, because often we ignore them, and they can have a cascade effect. Maybe when you wake up, "Dang it—we're out of coffee!" Then you go to feed the cats, "Dang it—we're out of cat food!" And then you trip and spill your breakfast all over the floor. All these little things start to add up through the day. If you can start to recognize the little things that really bother you, you may be able to do something, or take a break, before the stress starts cascading into something bigger. Or, we might notice that instead of ignoring the little things, we tightly hold onto them in our minds. "Oh boy, it's only 9:00 a.m., and all this stuff has happened—this is going to be a bad day!" So, we carry our irritation about this being a bad day around with us. Instead, we can practice something like, "Boy, this started off as a bad day. Let me take a breath, and let me take care of myself, and I can start fresh from this moment." So, we'll start with noticing what upsets us, so we'll have more conscious choices about what we want to do in the next moment, if anything.

All right, thanks everybody, and we'll see you next week!

8   Session 4

Recognizing Aversion

In the original MBCT protocol, this session was called "Staying Present." The new title highlights that we must first notice our habitual tendency to push away unpleasant experiences, which is what often keeps us locked into maladaptive patterns. Practicing mindfulness helps us gain a wider perspective on our experiences, opening up opportunities to relate differently to our difficulties. This session also brings more awareness to patterns of thinking, particularly in relation to challenges like depression and anxiety.

Of note, the revised edition does not include showing the *Healing From Within* video (Kabat-Zinn & Moyers, 1993). Zindel Segal told me that he felt it was no longer necessary (Segal & Lau, 2013). When mindfulness programs like MBCT were new, it was important to show that other people were doing this. However, the video can be hard to obtain, is now a bit dated, and might imply that the program is "Buddhist."

As you will see again in this session, it is important to be flexible in delivery of the program. When a question comes up about the usefulness of the course, I felt it important to address it directly before bringing the group back to processing the exercise. When significant feelings of sadness came up, and talk about death, it provided an opportunity to model staying present with difficult emotions rather than automatically avoiding them, which is the theme of this session.

Session 4 Transcript

Dr. Sears: All right—any burning questions or comments before we jump in with the exercise?

Kevin: I had a cool phrase occur to me during one of the times I was doing the sitting meditation. The phrase that came to me was, "I am open for 'isness.'"

Laura: For 'isness'?

Kevin: What do you think?

Christine: You'll get some laughs [laughter].

Dr. Sears: All right, let's open ourselves up for "isness" right now [laughter]. We're going to do a sitting meditation much like we did last week. We're just going to add one more thing on the end.

[Exercise—breath, body, working with difficult sensations, sounds, thoughts]

Dr. Sears: So what did people notice during that exercise?
Laura: I think it's challenging to look at your thoughts.
Dr. Sears: It is.
Laura: And to try and step back from them. I felt like I could see them, and then I was in them, and then I could see them, and then I was in them. It's almost like I had to be in them to even recognize that I was having a thought. It's challenging, but throughout the week, I found myself recognizing certain thoughts that I wouldn't have in the past, and specifically, things that would cause anxiety. I'm getting a little bit better at stepping back and looking.
Dr. Sears: That's wonderful. It's a pretty advanced skill to be able to see your own thoughts. So your experience is very typical. Even noticing that you're able to just sometimes step back is wonderful. And you'll immediately get pulled back in again, of course, but that's great that you're noticing that.
Other experiences?
Christine: I understand what mindfulness is, the concept, but how does that directly relate to stress reduction? I mean, we're not trying to breathe more deeply, we're just more aware of our breath. We're not trying to think more positive thoughts, we're just more aware of our thoughts.
Dr. Sears: Right.
Christine: If our thoughts are stress related, should we try to think more positive thoughts? I don't know. . .
Dr. Sears: That's a really important question. I'm glad you felt safe enough to ask that, because I don't want you to just go along and hope that maybe someday it sinks in, or that there's some hidden thing going on. One of our first goals is just to develop more awareness of what our patterns are, of what the mind's patterns are, what goes on in our body, how we react to things. And then, we can consciously choose to respond to what's happening, instead just reacting out of habit. Especially with stress, we get into these habits of thought. We may have running thought commentaries, and automatic thoughts that come up whenever certain situations happen. A lot of times, we're not even aware of these thoughts, kind of like background processing. Yet, these thoughts have a big impact on how we're feeling, as we talked about in session two. When you have a thought, that triggers a feeling, which triggers a thought, and so on, and you can get lost in those feelings and thoughts without knowing why. By learning to notice, "Wow, I'm having a lot of thoughts right now about failing," or pain, or whatever it is, I can kind of step back and notice that, and then I can recognize, "I'm having so many pressured thoughts—that

must mean I'm stressed." So then I can choose to take a break, to step away, or to come into my body. Because a lot of times, the thoughts are a way of distracting myself from the unpleasant feelings that I'm having. By coming back into the body, I can feel the feeling, and then it will be more likely to wash through, and then will be less overwhelming.

So, in a way, there is a little bit of a faith piece to this, a bit of trust that this is all going to come together. We have to start with just noticing where we are to begin with, and noticing when stress is coming up in the body. For a lot of us, we don't even notice tension is building, the stress is building, the pain is building, our resistance is building, until we're overwhelmed, so now the goal is to just notice it's starting to build up. And if you're talking about anxiety, or panic, or depression, our typical pattern is, "I don't want to feel this—I'm going to pretend it's not there!" But if it is already here, I'm just going to notice it, and see what's happening, and observe it. Then, I can make a more conscious choice about what to do next, instead of falling into an automatic reaction that might have helped in the past, but may or may not be so helpful right now.

You asked a very good question. I hope you're all asking this of yourselves as we go along. "How can I use this? Where are we going with this?" Of course, in a sense, just being more present in our lives can be pretty rewarding, but I know all of you have some pretty serious life struggles going on too that you want to make sure you can be using this with. When we get to the home practice for today, you're going to be asked to start practicing with daily life stressors, using the three-minute breathing space whenever you notice you are getting distressed. This is one way we'll start to interrupt the old patterns we often get caught up in.

Christine: And so if we're feeling pain, should we try and relax our muscles, or should we just feel the pain? Should we make a conscious effort to think about things that are more positive, or just be more aware of that at this point?

Dr. Sears: You know, that's a really good question. Ultimately, it's going to come down to being more free to trust your own inner wisdom, as funny as that might sound at first. You'll notice, "Well, I'm in pain right now, but I've got to go to this board meeting, so I'm just going to try to push it down and ignore it." As a conscious choice, maybe that's what you decide. But if your habit is to push it down every time you feel it, that takes a lot of energy, and the tension and pain often builds up and builds up over time. So, you might be at home and notice it's hurting, and you might decide to sit with it for a minute, allowing it to be there as it is, exploring it, which allows you to learn to relate to it differently. When you practice this, over time, the tension eases up, and even if you still have pain, the sense of suffering will often diminish some. The funny thing about relaxation is that it's really hard to force yourself to relax. It tends to happen more naturally when you are just, "All right, this is how it is. Even though I don't like it, this is how it is." You learn to let go of some of the struggle.

Stephanie: You're full of tension.

Dr. Sears: Yes. You're full of tension. That's a good description. I was just talking to someone today who hadn't kayaked since she was a kid, and she's in her fifties now. So she's out there on the lake with a friend who's trying to coach her how to kayak, how to coordinate the paddle and everything. She said, "I was working so hard, and I just couldn't get it. I kept messing up." And she said, "The harder I tried, the more I just kept going in circles, which is an interesting life analogy." Her back and shoulders began hurting. At one point, she told herself, "I'm just going to stop trying so hard, and I'm just going to have fun!" She said immediately after that, it was just like magic. Her friend said, "That's it! You're doing it!" And then she was just flowing along smoothly, and had a great time.

That's an interesting analogy. If you're struggling with pain, or stress, or anxiety, or depression, it may not completely go away—suffering is a part of life. It's going to be there. But when you relate to it differently, and you let go of some of the struggle and the resistance, our lives can flow a little bit more freely.

Any other things about this exercise we just did? We did breath, and then feeling the body, and then sounds, and then thoughts.

Stephanie: I was aware of inner sadness. Just going through this divorce. Just "ughh."

Dr. Sears: Yeah, lots of sadness.

Stephanie: And then it was interesting, because I've got a corn on this toe, and it was like competing.

Dr. Sears: Oh, throbbing and grabbing your attention?

Stephanie: Yeah. So then it was like ping pong, with my attention bouncing back and forth.

Laura: Did you mean the pain in your toe and the sadness were competing with each other?

Stephanie: It kind of felt like that. Yeah. They were competing for my attention. It was kind of interesting. Different types of pain, but . . .

Dr. Sears: And what a wonderful attitude to have, to say "Isn't that interesting?" Many people would be like, "Damn! I'm sad, and on top of that, my foot is hurting!"

Stephanie: Well, I didn't want to be sad, and I was sitting here crying. So I was like, "Oh, well, shit." [laughter]

Laura: It gets better. The whole divorce thing.

Stephanie: We told our boys. And that was really hard. [crying]
Dr. Sears: That's always hard. So for you, sadness is here. To deny it, and push it down, is not going to make it any better.
Anything else come up for people?
Kevin: I was remarkably quiet, which felt great. I just came straight here from a meeting. After the meeting, making plans, arrangements, follow-ups, driving out here, moving pretty quickly. I was really happy with how quiet I could be.
Dr. Sears: Wonderful—it's hard to really let that go sometimes.
Kevin: Yeah. When you were asking us to observe our thoughts, I was able to sit through three cycles of in and out breaths with no thoughts occurring, which was really unusual for me, actually.
Dr. Sears: So you were aware of your breathing, and didn't notice any thoughts at first. When I said to look for your thoughts, did anyone notice it was hard to find them, almost as if your mind went clear? That is fairly common.
Laura: The whole visualizing them doesn't work for me.
Dr. Sears: Okay.
Laura: The leaves and the clouds. I don't know. I can't see them like that.
Dr. Sears: Everyone's going to be different in how they perceive thoughts. I try to be careful, because sometimes I can say something like that, and then everyone thinks, "Well, I've got to do it that way." But it's very individualized, how you experience your own thoughts. Images are meant to be metaphors to help you get started, but can actually get in the way of noticing the thoughts directly.
Laura: It was weird, because with the recording, one time it did work. I imagined them as leaves. But now it doesn't.
Dr. Sears: That's fine. You can just try one of the metaphors, and if it's not working, you can try something else, or just drop them altogether. They're only meant to be tools to help you notice thoughts more clearly.
I think there's another interesting phenomenon worth discussing. Have you ever had the experience where you can't stop thinking about something?
Everyone: Oh, yeah.
Dr. Sears: When you get better at this, you can see that as a sign. "Okay, I'm noticing I'm thinking about this a lot, so it must mean that I'm distressed or upset." So you can then choose to feel the distress in your body, and that kind of undercuts the need, the pressure to think, because the compulsive thinking is serving to distract you from the feeling of distress in your body.
The other thing you can do is just notice and watch the thoughts, rather than getting caught up in them. Again, it's the opposite of trying not to think about it. "I'm trying not to think about this, but the thoughts aren't stopping. Okay, I'm just going

to look at you." And the more you do that, the more you discover that it's actually hard to hold on to a thought. You'll start to see that it breaks up. Just like pain. It kind of breaks up when you stay present with it. It comes and goes. And it's usually not as scary as you feared it would be when you were trying to not think of the thoughts.

Stephanie: I noticed that when you asked us to take our attention away from our breath to the sounds, that as I was listening to the sounds, I realized that I wasn't breathing anymore. I thought, "I better breathe." And then when you were just talking about that, as far as thoughts, a couple of years ago, I was having some fear-based issues. I was seeing a therapist at the time, and he suggested that whenever I had fear, that I just really focus on it. Be in a safe place, and really focus on it, and it's amazing how it really dissolves. I've really taken that with me whenever I'm really afraid of something. I'll sit down and really give it my attention, and it gets clearer, and I just also know what I need to do, if that makes sense. If it's not a real fear, there's just no getting my mind around it.

Dr. Sears: Now that's a great description of mindfulness. I'm just going to sit with this. How much of this is real? If I need to do something, and take some real action, then I'll be in a better place to do so if I first sit with it. Or is this just my mind going round and round, or old stuff that I can let go of? You can choose from a wiser place instead of automatically reacting.

Stephanie: There's a book called *The Gift of Fear*.

Dr. Sears: I haven't read it yet, but I heard good things about it. It's been on my bookshelf for a long time.

Stephanie: It's got a couple of really good stories in it. It's just fascinating. Fascinating.

Laura: That kind of reminds me of something I used to do when I was a teenager. I would often ask somebody if this was a healthy thing to do, or an unhealthy thing to do. I would have a thought of something that would make me sad, like imagining my parents dying. Usually it was when I was lying in bed thinking. I would allow myself to imagine, and I would allow myself to feel the sadness. And then I would cry. And then it would be gone. Is that normal? Is that a good thing to do?

Dr. Sears: It certainly can be a good thing to do. And in fact, there are Eastern traditions with a series of meditations where you begin to let go of your fear of death by imagining your own body decomposing and dying, and every loved one you have dying, and contemplating that you don't know when or how you will die—at the next breath, or fifty years from now. At first it sounds like a terrible idea to do that.

Stephanie: Like it would spark a panic attack!

Dr. Sears: But by staying with it, you have the experience that you did. You feel it, and then it settles, and the idea of death loses its sting. You feel much more free, and more appreciative of the moments and the relationships you do have left.

Laura: It almost felt like, by doing that, I could imagine myself handling it. And then my parents both did die while I was in my twenties. And then I felt, I mean, it was incredibly sad.

Dr. Sears: Of course.

Laura: And I went on depression medicines. And even when . . .

Stephanie: Your parents both died when you were in your twenties?

Laura: Yeah, I was 26 when my mom died, and 29 when my dad died.

Stephanie: Wow. It was like the universe was helping you prepare for that ahead of time.

Laura: I think it did, to imagine it ahead of time, to imagine dealing with it. And even when it did happen, I was incredibly sad . . .

Stephanie: Absolutely.

Laura: But I never felt like I was going to completely fall apart.

Dr. Sears: Yeah.

Laura: I mean, I had times when I felt like I was going to cry and be really sad . . .

Dr. Sears: Of course.

Laura: . . . but I never felt like my life was completely shattered.

Stephanie: Wow.

Dr. Sears: And that's why these traditions practice these kinds of meditations, because otherwise, for a lot of people, it just completely shatters their whole lives when something tragic happens that they were trying to avoid thinking was a possibility.

Stephanie: I want to ask another question regarding that, because if we're afraid of someone dying, and we're with that sadness, and we really give it our full attention, we're able to be with that person while they're still here in a more. . . .

Dr. Sears: Yes. That's another benefit. Because you've been there in your mind, and you've moved through the anxiety and avoidance, then what a gift it is to spend time with them.

Stephanie: Then you're not seeing things through that fear of losing them.

Dr. Sears: Yeah, you don't take them for granted quite so much. You recognize that none of us are going to live forever, so you're going to appreciate the interactions a little bit more.

Stephanie: That's cool. Thanks for sharing that.

Kevin: Speaking of parents and mortality, one of the reasons I'm here now, as long as I've been, is I've ended up kind of care taking for my parents. I'm based overseas, and this was just going to be a three-week visit for me. Mother, she's 83. Short-term memory is largely gone, so she repeats herself a lot. And one of the things she keeps repeating—talk about always having to deal with the fact of

	mortality—she loves to say, "Just think what you're going to get when we die," and she loves to state a dollar figure.
Laura:	She says that?
Kevin:	She says that. She probably says it 5–10 times a day.
Stephanie:	Oh my goodness.
Laura:	Is she trying to make you see a positive side about her dying?
Kevin:	It gives her great joy.
Laura:	Oh, well that's cool!
Kevin:	"Just think, you're going to get this much." It might not even be true really [laughter]. Who knows, really. But in her mind, there's this fixed amount that each of her kids is going to get. And it brings her great joy.
Laura:	Well, she's taking care of her kids!
Kevin:	Totally. There's nothing that brings her greater joy than giving to her kids. But I don't like hearing it. Psychologically. It's not something you like to hear, right? It's weird to think about it.
Christine:	Yeah, if it's repeated over and over, that gets kind of weird.
Kevin:	And a couple of times I've reacted. "Mom, I don't want to hear it!"
Laura:	Is it because you don't want her to concentrate on money, or because you don't want to think about her dying?
Kevin:	Yeah, each time she says it, it's bringing up the fact of her dying.
Dr. Sears:	And of course for her, with the short-term memory loss, it's the first time she's said it. So she doesn't have the sense that you do of it being repeated.
Kevin:	That's right.
Dr. Sears:	So, how about the home practice for the week? How did that go? The sitting meditation, walking or yoga, the three-minute breathing space, the unpleasant events calendar?
Laura:	I wasn't very consistent in doing it. But I was more consistent earlier in the week, and I felt like I was less stressed earlier in the week.
Dr. Sears:	Oh, okay.
Laura:	And then yesterday, I had a bad day, and I didn't do any of the stuff. And then I thought, "Well, maybe I should have done it!"
Dr. Sears:	Yeah. It's funny, right in the manual for this program, it says it's common to feel like now the honeymoon is over. About this time in the group, the newness and the freshness is wearing off, and you realize this is going to take some work and discipline. I find that if you just sit down, whether you "feel like it" or not, you can usually get right into the flow of it. Even at least noticing the resistance to doing it can be a practice. Just noticing what is going on with me, and even just practicing in that moment.
Kevin:	I did it quite detailed through the week, and then I gave myself the weekend off [laughter].

Christine: When I did the unpleasant events one, I tried to turn it into something positive, just because I'm a cause-and-effect person. I like to try to do something after I'm uncomfortable or in pain. Just noticing that my muscles are tight in reaction to whatever it is that happened helps me be able to try to relax a little bit. Noticing that if I've got pain because of something, to try and relax to reduce that. And also, things that have happened that are negative, I try to at least put a positive spin on it at the end of the day.

Dr. Sears: Yeah. Actually, that reminds me of when you asked that question about what do you do, as far as stress reduction. That's definitely an option. So the first step is noticing what is happening. Am I feeling stressed? Am I feeling pain? And then you can choose, "Do I want to think about this in a different way? Do I want to just stay with it? Do I just need to go on to something else?" It becomes more of a choice. And certainly replacing it with a more positive thought that feels natural and appropriate, is wonderful, as long as it's not always done out of avoidance.

I just saw a movie called *Happy*. They talk to researchers and different people about what contributes to happiness. It's a very interesting documentary. One of the things they talked about was a study that showed you increased your happiness if, once a week, you thought about just five things you are grateful for. And again, not forcing yourself, or making it artificial, but genuinely appreciating the things that are going well. Our brains have a tendency to always go towards the negative, because we need to fix and prevent problems. If it's positive, our brains often ignore it and move on to find the next problem. So, as you said, it can be a good exercise to remind ourselves of what we do have.

Anything else about the homework?

Stephanie: I don't think I did a very good job. I started out well, but . . . And I think part of it is, I'm just putting up blocks, and I'm putting up resistance. And whenever I do stop to pay attention to what's going on, I don't always like what is going on. And I'm going to put this handout on a place that doesn't get covered up on my desk.

Dr. Sears: And you know, it's got to be balanced. Consistency is very important, but you've also got to be kind to yourself.

Stephanie: And I'm trying not to beat myself up. I was even thinking about not coming tonight. "No, I'm going to go. I'm recommitting."

Dr. Sears: Recommitting is a good attitude. Getting caught up in guilt about past "failures" adds more baggage. Just start fresh in this moment. If you haven't been consistent on the homework, start over right now.

Kevin: I really like listening to the meditations.

Dr. Sears: Well, good. All right, one of our themes today is becoming more aware of our own thoughts. So, just to start to recognize that we can step back and notice that these thoughts are going to come and go, and to notice that we can start to recognize that there is often a pattern to them. And especially when you're stressed, anxious, depressed, or in pain, certain patterns of thinking will likely show up.

Here in the handout, we have an "automatic thoughts questionnaire." You don't have to fill this out necessarily. It's meant to be an example. The ones listed here are pretty common thoughts for individuals struggling with depression. When you see thoughts on a list as signs of stress, anxiety, or depression, you shift your relationship to them. In other words, we normally feel overly identified and stuck inside a thought like, "I am worthless." This may sound like semantics, but it can be a really powerful shift to realize, "Oh, I am having a thought that I am worthless. That means that I am starting to get depressed. I better go take care of myself, and do something for myself." Being able to see these thoughts down on paper helps you to recognize them, and kind of distance yourself from them when they do come up.

Stephanie: Kind of breaks them down.

Dr. Sears: Yeah. And that's one of the reasons journaling is so helpful. You're getting it out on paper. You're seeing it. It's now separate from you. We are not our thoughts, we *have* thoughts. We are not our feelings, we *have* feelings. We're the context in which those happen. Who we are is bigger than that.

On the left side of the automatic thoughts questionnaire, there's a frequency column, how often you have that thought. Chances are, if you're feeling depressed, you're going to have those thoughts more often. So, that can be a sign to you that you're feeling more and more depressed.

The right side column is degree of belief. It's possible some of these thoughts come up often, like "I'm worthless," but I recognize, "Oh, that's old stuff from my childhood. I don't really believe that anymore." Versus, when you're really depressed, and you really believe that you're worthless. Degree of belief can be an indicator of how depressed you are too.

You can start to make your own "negative thought hit parade." What are the top 10 thoughts I get when I'm depressed? When you learn to recognize them, instead of fighting them, you can take action to take care of yourself.

When this group program was originally studied, it caught a lot of scientific attention because it cut relapse rates for depression in half. Once you've been depressed, you're more likely to get depressed again, jumping up to an almost 80% chance once you've been depressed three or more times. Even once-a-month therapy or drugs aren't always helpful in preventing future episodes of depression.

We believe this group helps because we learn to pay more attention to the oncoming warning signs, so we can be proactive. Typically, when depression is coming back, it's so awful, you just don't want to feel it. You want to pretend that it's not really happening. You want to isolate yourself. You don't feel like doing anything, and stay home more. You cut yourself off from your social support. It's the opposite of noticing. All of this only makes the depression worse.

After practicing mindfulness, we can make a shift. "I am noticing I'm having depressive thoughts. I am noticing I'm withdrawing more. Even though I don't feel like doing it, I know I better get out more, and talk to friends more, and get more active." I can make a more conscious choice. It's much easier to pull yourself out of depression when you're just starting to slide down than when you're way down in it.

Same with stress and anxiety. I notice when I'm starting to get stressed. "I'm having these thoughts that I really want to ram into these drivers that are cutting me off. Oh boy, I usually don't have that thought, and drivers cut people off every day. So, it must mean that I'm getting stressed out. I better do something to prevent myself from getting more and more stressed out." If you don't notice it until it gets to the point where you're overwhelmed, it's much harder to deal with.

Laura: How is depression defined? It seems like there would be a real grey area where you're kind of depressed, but not to a point where you would be clinically. Is there a solid definition of it?

Dr. Sears: It's all on a continuum, of course, but I have the diagnostic criteria for major depressive disorder right here. One of the big pieces is that it lasts at least two weeks. So it's not just . . .

Stephanie: I was going to say, I know I'm sad from this divorce, and that's kind of normal and all, but I didn't think I was depressed . . .

Dr. Sears: And that's a normal reaction, based on your circumstances and all.

Kevin: And that was just one of the first criteria.

Dr. Sears: Five or more of these nine areas here, continuously over at least a two-week period. And it's a departure from normal, of course. This is not just feeling down for a few days. You literally can't pull yourself out of it with willpower—it's like you're physically sick. Feeling generally sad for most of the day. You lose your ability to feel pleasure, even from things you used to enjoy—the technical term is called anhedonia. Actually, I remember when I was going through my own divorce, thinking I would pull myself out of it with some comedy movies that used to make me really laugh out loud. I remember watching them and just not really feeling anything. That ability to feel pleasure is really diminished.

Stephanie: I could really go into a depression, though, if I don't let this sadness out, and stuff it all down, right?

Dr. Sears: You could, yeah. There are a lot of factors, though.

Stephanie: That's interesting.

Dr. Sears: Significant weight change, increase or decrease in appetite nearly every day. Difficulty sleeping through the night, or a need for more sleep during the day. For many, they're really tired when they fall sleep, and then they wake up at 3:00 or so in the morning and can't get back to sleep again. Noticeably slowed down or agitated throughout the day. Feeling fatigued, a loss of energy every day. Feelings of worthlessness, or extreme or inappropriate guilt. Difficulty concentrating, thinking, and making decisions. Thinking a lot about death and/or suicide. So those are the diagnostic criteria (American Psychiatric Association, 2000).

Laura: Thank you.

Dr. Sears: Sometimes I read the diagnostic criteria for people who are going through it, so they don't think, "It's just me." No, this is what happens when you're depressed, and you've gone through this life circumstance, and your brain chemistry, thinking, and behavior has gotten caught in this downward spiral pattern. This is just what depression is, or anxiety is, or whatever the diagnosis. And so, knowing this helps you take it less personally. You can recognize, "'I'm a failure' is a thought. That's not me, that is the disease of depression." Now I can work on the underlying issue, recovering from the depression, which requires becoming more active, rather than getting stuck in battling my own thoughts.

Laura: Is anxiety similar, or is that completely different?

Dr. Sears: Interestingly, they can often be comorbid, meaning you can fully have both, or you can have one with aspects of the other. So with depression can come some anxiety, or if you get overwhelmed with a lot of anxiety you can start to get a little depression in there too. I don't have my diagnostic manual with me, but there are of course lists of criteria for the anxiety disorders. When I'm teaching my doctoral students about diagnosis, one of the most important things I want them to remember is that we're all on a continuum. So, if the depression or anxiety gets to the point where it's interfering with your life and your ability to function, that's when we consider a diagnosis, but some degree of anxiety or depression is part of the normal human experience. This group helps us by teaching us to recognize sooner the buildup of depression, anxiety, stress, or other problems so we can take action before they become overwhelming.

Laura: Thank you.

Dr. Sears: So, the theme for today is staying present. You can read through this in the handout later, but typically, we have three different ways we react to our experiences. Sometimes we're just unaware—we might kind of "space out" a little bit, or feel bored and go off in our heads somewhere and not really be present. Or, if we really like something, we might really want to hold on to it. We want it to last forever. Have you ever had that experience? You're enjoying it, but then you become self-conscious because you really don't want it to end, and are not as fully in the experience because you're really trying to grab on to it. The other thing we often do automatically is try to push away what we don't want. If we are doing these three things continuously, it takes a lot of energy. Another option is to consciously choose to stay present with our experiences as they already are in the moment we are in.

This is not necessarily about labeling these three tendencies as "good" or "bad." Be careful about developing a new set of "shoulds." "I should not want this." "I should not want to push it away." "I should be more present." The whole idea is to start with noticing what you're doing.

I'm laughing because there was a therapist named Albert Ellis who really liked to play with words and say "Don't should all over yourself!" [laughter]. All these expectations of what you have to do. The idea is to be more present and to notice. "I'm noticing I really want to hold onto this, and of course I want to hold onto this, because it feels really good! But I can just enjoy it for what it is right now."

After all, mental tension, whether of grabbing or pushing away, does not change the reality—it only wears us out or distracts us from the moment. I remember when I was working in a cornfield as a teenager, and I found some beautiful morning glory flowers. I pulled one off to enjoy it, and it literally withered up in my hand. Had I left it as it was, I would have enjoyed it longer. While I'm thinking about how to possess an experience, I am not present in the moment with it as fully.

So, we're going to practice just staying present with our experiences more often. And again, it doesn't mean you have to like what's happening. What comes up could be awful. It could be pain. It could be sadness. "I don't like this. I don't want it to be here. But it's here. I can't push it away. I'm just going to notice that it's here." When you stay with it, it tends to break up and change. If you fight it too much, you add extra energy, and feel sad about the sadness, feel pain about the pain, or feel anxious about the anxiety. When we struggle with ourselves, we add a lot of extra suffering.

Okay, I'm going to go ahead and get the video ready. Any questions or comments while the projector is warming up? This video is actually a little bit dated—it's from 1990.

Session 4: Recognizing Aversion 129

Laura: It's funny to me to think about 1990 as being old [laughter].
Dr. Sears: Right—my glasses were big like the ones in the video not all that long ago [laughter]. This video shows Jon Kabat-Zinn leading a group of people through an eight-week mindfulness-based stress reduction course, so you can see some experiences that others have had.

[First half of *Healing From Within* video]

Dr. Sears: We'll watch the second half next week. Any questions or comments?
Kevin: What's that journalist's name?
Dr. Sears: Bill Moyers.
Christine: Is that who that was?
Dr. Sears: Yeah, that came from a PBS series called *Healing and the Mind*.
Stephanie: That was really good.
Laura: I liked the part about the chatter of the mind.
Stephanie: It's amazing how foreign it was back then.
Laura: But aren't some people still resistant to it?
Dr. Sears: I think so, but not as much as it used to be. I actually have a friend who owns a martial arts school who said he got put on "cult watch" when he offered a meditation class a couple of years ago.
Kevin: That's a remarkable individual. You can just tell.
Dr. Sears: Oh, Jon Kabat-Zinn? Yeah. He's great.
   Before we look at the home practice, let's do a three-minute breathing space.

[Exercise—3-minute breathing space]

Dr. Sears: What did you notice about that exercise?
Laura: That went really fast. That was three minutes?
Dr. Sears: Actually, that was a little shorter. In fact, as you practice dropping into the moment more often, you might even experiment with doing three breaths instead of three minutes.
   The first part of the homework is to continue to do the sitting meditation: breath, body, sounds, and thoughts. The second part is to again keep practicing the three-minute breathing space three times a day. Continue to do it as an exercise at set times.
   And the third part is to do what we call the "three-minute breathing space—responsive." All that means is, can you notice during the day when you're feeling distressed, and remember to pause and do this three-minute breathing space? The idea is to remember to notice what you're experiencing, rather than automatically pushing through and ignoring things like stress. Don't even expect that you're going to do this to make yourself feel better, just check in with how you are in that moment. Just do it as an experiment.
Christine: How is listening to the sounds part of all this? Is that just practicing more awareness?

Dr. Sears: Yes—you can use any of your senses. In fact, Jon Kabat-Zinn wrote a book called *Coming to Our Senses*. It helps us get more into the moment instead of living in our heads.

And the last thing is, if you want to learn more about Jon Kabat-Zinn and the program he developed, you might want to read his book, *Full Catastrophe Living*. Another one of his books is called *Wherever You Go, There You Are*. It has very short chapters, so it's nice to read a little of it at a time to inspire you to keep practicing after the course is over.

Christine: If you have a short attention span.
Stephanie: I actually have that book.
Dr. Sears: All right, thanks for coming!

9 Session 5
Allowing/Letting Be

In this session, we practice intentionally allowing things to be exactly as we find them in the moment, even if what we discover is unpleasant. This involves the development of a sense of kindness toward ourselves and our experiences, letting go of the struggles and judgments we get caught up in with our own thoughts, feelings, and sensations. When we can see things more clearly, we can make better decisions about what we can do in the next moment, if anything.

In this session and in the next two, we ask clients to purposefully sit with a difficulty, and if one is not already present, to bring one to mind. It can be challenging for new therapists to do this, as we are trained to help clients feel better, not ask them to feel worse. Training in and understanding of exposure therapy can be helpful. Though it can be hard to gauge with a room full of diverse participants, it is ideal to allow enough time for people to observe changes in how they experience the difficulty. As with exposure work, remind them to stay present with the difficulty they have chosen. Every time the mind goes off to something else, the exposure process is basically starting over again.

Mindful inquiry is particularly important here, as this is a profound turning point in the course for many. I explicitly ask the group, "You came here to feel better. Why would we practice bringing something difficult to mind on purpose?" Most will recognize that when they stayed present with something they were trying to avoid, they had trouble doing so, or they became more aware of how they were reacting to it, or were able to separate the situation from the thoughts, emotions, and body sensations that came up. In almost every case, participants will say that the experience was not as bad as they "thought" it would be.

Importantly, even if clients say they did not feel "better" by the end of the exercise, they have learned that they can choose to sit with something difficult without becoming completely overwhelmed by it. I once had someone say they felt "worse" when the exercise ended, but during inquiry, when I asked how she was feeling now, she realized the strong feelings had passed. Experiencing the fact that unpleasant thoughts, emotions, and sensations change and pass away even when we do not "do something" about them is very powerful.

Session 5 Transcript

Dr. Sears: Any burning questions or thoughts before we get started?

Stephanie: I don't know if it's because in our meditations we've been focusing more on the hearing, but I've just been more aware of hearing different things, different noises. In fact, after our class last week, I kept hearing something in my house. I ran out to see if it was outside. I think I was just more attuned to the water going through the pipes or something. It was interesting.

Dr. Sears: Yeah.

Laura: Paying more attention to that kind of stuff.

Dr. Sears: I think like most of our senses, until something big grabs our attention, we don't notice very often. The other thing we were talking about too is that your mind gets quieter, so it's easier to hear more of what's going on.

All right, any big questions before we jump in with our exercise? All right, let's take a moment to settle in from the rush of getting here. We're going to start off like we did last week, and we're just going to add one more thing on at the end.

[Exercise—sitting meditation. Breath, body, sounds, thoughts, introducing a difficulty]

Dr. Sears: All right, what did people notice during that exercise? We did quite a few different things in there.

Stephanie: When you had us focus on the unpleasant or uncomfortable, I thought of a person that I feel kind of slighted me. Well, not slighted me, avoided me. Well, not avoided me, is just not making an effort to be in contact, and it's been bugging me. And so I just focused on that, but it was interesting. The more I focused on that, I had a peace, and I even had like a tingling sensation, like I have a comfort that it's going to be okay.

Dr. Sears: Mmmm. How interesting.

Stephanie: It was interesting. Because it wasn't the result that I thought, which was, "Oh, no, I'm going to cry again!"

Dr. Sears: I often find that to be the case. It's such an automatic thing to push away what we don't like or don't want to feel. We can just say, "Okay, I'm just going to feel it." Usually it does get worse at first, but if we stay with it long enough, it tends to change.

Stephanie: In a way, it's like I'm getting myself worked up into a tizzy over something that's not tizzy qualified.

Laura: Not tizzy worthy [laughter].

Stephanie: Exactly!
Dr. Sears: Right. And again, there could be some situations that require a tizzy [laughter]. But you can decide for yourself how much is tied into what's really happening, and how much is tied up into something else. We often don't know until we sit with it.
Stephanie: That was a surprise.
Dr. Sears: Well, good.
Kevin: I like that tingle you're talking about. It doesn't happen often. Just rarely. But when it tingles, that tingle is "isness." That tingle is, you're right there. You're right in the moment.
Dr. Sears: That's interesting.
Laura: I kept wanting to try and figure out a solution for the difficult situation.
Dr. Sears: Okay.
Christine: I'm the same way. If there's a problem, I want to try and find a solution and do something about it. I struggle with it when you say, "Let's focus on pain." I want to do something about it.
Dr. Sears: Yeah.
Laura: I don't know. What can you do?
Dr. Sears: So what happened in this exercise? You noticed you wanted to fix it, or maybe you were thinking of ways to fix it. Were you able to come back and stay with it again, even if very briefly?
Laura: Kind of. My issue that I focused on is my financial situation. The recession has hit my practice, and we're very up and down, and I can't predict how we're going to do. There are some things I can do about it, and there are some things I have no control over. So when I was focusing on it, I felt like I can't think about it all the time, because there aren't things I can do about it all the time.
Dr. Sears: Right.
Laura: It's hard to just be with the situation now, and not try and figure out what's going to happen in the future.
Dr. Sears: Yeah.
Christine: I have the same issue. I have the same situation, where it feels like I've just lost control over the situation, and I think that's why I want to find a solution, because I feel like I don't have any control over things.
Dr. Sears: Right.
Christine: It helps if you can have a plan or something.
Laura: Yeah, and there's sometimes when you can plan, and then there's parts of it you can't.
Dr. Sears: Yeah. And this was just a one-time, "take a look at this." This is pretty advanced really, and it takes some practice to just allow something difficult to be present as it is, without making it worse. Of course, we want to think out solutions and we want to fix

things. But sometimes it becomes compulsive. I can't help it. I'm thinking about it all the time. I'm not paying attention to the person I'm with. I'm not enjoying myself. It's just this constant chatter running in the background. At a subtle level, maybe I don't want to feel the distress, so I'm going to try and think about how to fix it. But while I'm busy thinking about it, I'm also going to try and push it away, which often can make it a little bit worse. So, it's important to watch how we respond internally to difficulties. To just notice that I might have a choice. Sometimes I can sit with it, and perhaps let it pass. Sometimes, I really do want to think about it and take some action.

In fact, a therapy technique when you are really stuck, and can't stop thinking about something, is to tell yourself, "Okay, at seven o'clock tonight, when I'm at home and no one's around, that's when I'm going to worry." Especially when the thoughts start to get intrusive, and you can't concentrate, and you're always distracted. It's like a little trick to tell yourself that you will still worry about it, just not all day long. And sure enough, at 7 p.m., you should sit down and say, "Okay, I'm going to worry now."

Stephanie: And just really focus on it.

Dr. Sears: Yeah. Let it be there. Sit with it. Now what's funny to me is how often people say, "When 7 p.m. came around, I forgot to worry!" [laughter]. But it gives yourself permission to let it go, knowing you can worry later. It counters the thought, "I gotta fix this now, or when else will I do it?", which could turn into a compulsion. If it's just circular, if you're just thinking the same things over and over, it's not really thinking it through and fixing it. So it can be better to decide, "Okay, right now I want to sit down and have a cup of coffee, and just think about this problem," versus just carrying it all day long.

Stephanie: Well, during the meditation, didn't you ask us just to look at it without trying to fix it, or without trying to change it?

Dr. Sears: Yeah, just as it is.

Stephanie: Just as it is. It was interesting, because at one point I remembered something that happened today. I went walking around the Nature Center with a friend. And as we were walking, and we were walking fast, all of a sudden I looked down, and there at my feet I found 20 dollars. So I picked it up, and I thought, "Wow, this meditating thing is really paying off!"

Kevin: It's really paying off literally!

Laura: You seriously found 20 dollars?

Stephanie: I did! Then I picked it up, and I immediately felt guilty. And I thought, "No, I'm not guilty of anything. I found 20 dollars." And then I wanted to give it to my friend. So I'm having this argument with myself. The universe gave me 20 dollars, and I'm having a

	hard time keeping it. It was hilarious. But that was something, just a gift literally at my feet. And sometimes I think with meditation, we can get those gifts too. We really can.
Dr. Sears:	Yeah. It's amazing how much we really just don't notice.
Kevin:	I had an interesting similar situation today.
Laura:	You found 20 dollars too!
Kevin:	No, I found 10!
Laura:	No way! Damn, where's my money? [laughter]
Kevin:	But in a different way. We had to get this carpet in our bathroom dry cleaned. So I brought it to a dry cleaner. And in my mind, it was a 10-dollar job. So I called them later to ask how much they were going to charge to clean it. And they said 20 dollars. I asked the other people involved, and they said yeah, it's worth 20 dollars, go ahead and let them clean it. So I said, "It's your choice—it's your money." So today, we came to pick it up. And it was like 21 dollars and 10 cents with tax. So I look at my wallet, and I have a 20, but I don't have a one. So I tell her I don't have a one. So she says, "Oh, that's all right, $20.02 will be fine. So she takes $20.02, and she gives me back 10 dollars by mistake [laughter]. And I accepted it, because I thought the job was worth 10 dollars to begin with. So she confirmed that.
Dr. Sears:	She was not quite as mindful [laughter].
Kevin:	She will be when she balances things out later! [laughter]
Dr. Sears:	So just learning to sit with things can be important. Even with pain. Like when you said, "I feel pain, and I want to fix it." That's natural. And certainly, sometimes you can do something, like sitting a different way, that will help. At other times, there may be nothing you can do, and obsessive thinking doesn't make it go away. Another option is, what if I just let it be what it is, and just feel it? It's probably going to get a little worse at first, and then it just changes and shifts. And that's important. The goal is not that I'm going to transform it all the time, but I just have one more way of dealing with a difficulty, which is to go into it instead of thinking about it or avoiding it.
Christine:	Usually if I'm aware of it, it gives me a chance to try and relax those muscles, which then helps with the pain. But if you're not mindful of it, then it's just going to be worse.
Dr. Sears:	Yeah, good example.
Kevin:	Yeah, I mean your focus for us for this past week was to try and apply that three-minute meditation at times of coping, at difficult times and. . .
Dr. Sears:	Let me just pause on that for a second—anything else about this exercise before we talk about the previous week? Because that was a good segue. No? Okay, go ahead.
Kevin:	Yeah, I would segue it into what we were just doing.

Dr. Sears: Okay.

Kevin: Because for me, my issue is anxiety. And not just, "Oh, I feel anxious." No, I mean real anxiety, like I have to get up and go out of the room at times. So I tried throughout the week when it was at its worst to try and do that three-minute exercise. And I kind of developed a system. I scored a ratio of attention versus nonattention. If I was just 100% with the breath the whole time it would be 100:0. If my thoughts were completely in control and I never came back once it would be 0:100. So I found pretty consistently that when I was really, really anxious and tried to do the exercise, the ratio would be like 25% attention, 75% inattention, you know.

Dr. Sears: Sure.

Kevin: Versus times when I was calmer, which tends to be later in the evening, which would be like 70:30. So I started to actually quantify it. And it helps me. And then I could look back and compare and say, "Hey, look at that—in the mornings you tend to be anxious." So when you were doing the exercise just now, my mind went to a training that I'll be conducting on Thursday morning. I've been back in town a couple of months. And because of the severity of the anxiety, and earlier of depressive symptoms, I haven't been able to work. This will be my first real paid gig since I've come back. And I used to do these trainings quite often. They're cross-cultural trainings for executives who are relocating from another country. So I used to be able to do them without even much preparation, because I was familiar with it and everything. But it's been quite a while. It's almost like doing it from scratch now. There's a tizzy. Definitely a tizzy. This one probably merits a tizzy. It's just a question of how tizzy do I have to get in order to do a decent job?

Dr. Sears: Yeah. I think that's important. It's just noticing, "This is where I'm at." Honestly, I was having some trouble focusing today, and I realized, "Well yeah, I worked all weekend." We had a National Faculty Meeting, so the last four days I've been working very long days. And I got up at 5:30 this morning, and I've been working all day. So yeah, my mind's just not as focused. So just noticing, "That's my experience right now." Noticing that. Otherwise, I might start to berate myself, "Oh, damn it, I'm only 25% focused." Twenty-five percent is actually pretty good. And the fact that you're aware of that will help guide your decision process. Given that, do I need to go take a break? Am I still okay to continue? Do I need to just sit here for a while? Just bringing more consciousness to what you want to do.

Good. Anything else about how the week went? Other experiences of using the three-minute breathing space as a practice in the middle of something stressful?

Session 5: Allowing/Letting Be **137**

Laura: I felt that if I was feeling stressed, it was at a point where I didn't have time for those three minutes, but I just tried to condense it down.
Dr. Sears: Oh good.
Laura: In a very short period of time. Just notice my breath, and where I was right then. Look at my own thoughts.
Dr. Sears: Uh-huh.
Laura: And then go on with what I needed to do.
Dr. Sears: How did that work for you?
Laura: It helps. It wasn't perfect, but it definitely helps.
Dr. Sears: Well, it will never be perfect [laughter]. In what way did you notice it helping? You relaxed?
Laura: Yeah. Less tension. Less anxiety.
Dr. Sears: Wonderful.
Stephanie: I feel like, with going through this divorce, I'm on an emotional roller coaster. There are times when I feel like, "So much hope! I'm going to be free! It's going to be great!" Then there are times when it's like, "Oh my gosh, I'm so tired of this!" There's this emotional up and down, up and down. But I noticed that when I did the three minutes, if I was in a really good spot, joy would grow. When I focused on the joy, the joy would get bigger, and there was more a sense of joy, and that was nice.
Dr. Sears: Yeah. Obviously, the ups and downs are natural for what you're going through. But it reminds me that sometimes we're afraid we might lose a feeling of joy, so there's a weird relationship to the joy……
Stephanie: This too will pass.
Dr. Sears: I'm going to feel it, and this is here right now, instead of really getting caught up in trying to hold onto it so it doesn't go away, and strangling it [laughter].
Stephanie: Well it was funny, because there was a friend that had texted me, and I had gone to a meeting, and he had asked me how I was doing. I said, "I'm really doing well right here, right now." Then he texted me and said "I'm really glad you're doing well." And I replied back and said "thank you." Well, almost a day later, he replied back and said "you're welcome," but I was like, "I was full of joy then—I'm not full of joy now!" [laughter]. Boy, a lot can change in 15 hours!
Dr. Sears: And it will change again.
Stephanie: Yes, it will.
Kevin: I had one of those "you can't hold onto the moment even though you'd like to" moments today, when the car I was driving changed. I looked down at the speedometer—I don't know why I looked down at it—and the speedometer was at exactly 50,000 miles. Perfect 50,000. So clingy [laughter].
Laura: A little OCD moment.
Dr. Sears: All lined up.

Kevin: It was perfect! And I thought, "Wow, that is really beautiful."

Christine: Did you take a picture of it? [laughter]

Kevin: And I let it go. I'm going to be able to enjoy this for some fraction of a mile. I can't hold onto it. It's going to change to 1 at any second now. I can't hold onto that 50,000. So I enjoyed it while it was on there, and when it went to 1, I said, "okay" [laughter].

Stephanie: It's the little things.

Kevin: Little things. That's exactly what life is. The little things.

Christine: I had a question about the sounds. I don't find that to be helpful. I have a lot of hypersensitivity to sounds, and smells, and temperature, and light. I notice sounds when I don't want to. I don't want to hear all the sounds that I do. And I don't want to smell every smell. I smell things other people don't pick up on, just because I'm more sensitive. What is the reason—is it just being more aware of your surroundings?

Dr. Sears: Yeah, just to recognize that you can do mindfulness with any of your senses. So we started with the body because it's the most concrete. But you can do it with what you're looking at—20 dollars [laughter]. You can do it with sounds or smells. The raisin, the taste of your food. It's just that those are concrete things that are happening now. Your senses are what's happening now. Your thinking tends to be a little removed from your experiences. The only way you can experience anything in the world is through your senses. So, on the one hand, whatever practice feels best to you might be your gateway to getting more in touch with the present moment. And if it works for you, then that's great.

The other thing I would say is, there might be something important there if it's difficult. Because there are always sounds going on. It's not the sounds, it's our reactions to them. This is true for all of us. We all have different reactions to some sight, or some sound, or some smell, or some memory, or some thought. So, what we're working on is exploring, "What is this reaction all about?" It could just be that you're wired differently, and you notice there's a strong brain signal or whatever. So you can just watch that. But what can happen is, that strong signal comes in, and just as my muscles can tighten around the pain, my mind can tighten around a sound, a sight, or a thought. I just start to recognize, "Hmmm, I'm noticing this about myself." I may be able to find some way to relate differently to it. Or it could just be, "No, this is how I'm wired," and I get medical advice about it, or I just choose to avoid noisy places. It's about more awareness, and trying to decide what is best for you.

Christine: Thank you.

Dr. Sears: So the theme for today is about "allowing and letting be." This is what we were getting at with bringing the difficulty into the meditation. Can you just allow it to be there? You can read this over later in the handout, but the part that says that acceptance is not resignation is very important. "Acceptance, as a vital first step, allows us to become fully aware of difficulties, and then, if appropriate, to *respond* in a skillful way rather than to *react* in knee-jerk fashion, by automatically running off some of our old (often unhelpful) strategies for dealing with difficulties" (Segal, Williams, & Teasdale, 2002, p. 240). If I could only have one paragraph to describe the point of this whole course, that's probably the one I'd pull out. Just to accept that in this moment, this is just how it is. In the next moment, I can choose how I want to respond consciously, rather than with an automatic reaction like, "I hate it! I hate you! I can't stand this!", or with a reaction like, "I've got to hold on to it, or I'm gonna die! I've got to squeeze it to death!" Here it is, as it is. I might like it. I might not like it. I'm a little more aware of my impulses and reactions. I'm a little more aware of the choices I have in this moment. I can choose more freely. And again, the goal is not necessarily to do this 100% of the time. That would just wear us out. But even just once in a while, a little more often, just noticing, "Oh, I'm about to do something automatically again. Is this best for this situation?"

And what's fascinating to me is how often people come in here and notice that their relationships begin to change, whether with a partner, or with friends, or whomever. Because—if I can use you as an example?

Stephanie: Sure.

Dr. Sears: Something happens with someone you know, and your perception of it creates a feeling. We all can relate to that. "I don't like how this person looked at me," or "What they said rubbed me the wrong way," so I distance myself from them. And then, they begin thinking, "Well, that person's cold! I'm not going to talk to them anymore!", and the next thing you know I have this self-fulfilling prophecy. What can happen in this course is people begin to notice and let go of automatic reactions, and then they're more open. Because they're less defensive, the people they are talking to are less defensive, and they feel closer, and then spend more time together, and their relationships get better.

We can really get so pulled in to old reactions. You may feel a strong urge to tell someone off, but you might realize, "It's just not going to help right now. It's just going to make me look out of control. I'm just going to let it go." Or you might decide, "This is so important, I need to set strong boundaries." I more often recognize the choices I have, even if my feelings are strong.

Laura: It was interesting. I had something happen recently. I have a really close friend, and he has a girlfriend he's been dating for a while. He was telling me that she was unhappy with me about something. And in the past, this would have *really* bothered me. I would have really gotten upset about this. So, I was like, "Okay, I get she's interpreting something I did maybe not in the best way." And it surprised me that I didn't get upset about it. Before, it would have really bothered me.

Dr. Sears: Good!

Stephanie: Cool!

Laura: So I just continued to interact with her the same way that I always have. Time will tell if she stays upset with me or not.

Dr. Sears: And again, that's a great attitude for mindfulness. "I can't control how she reacts, but I can control what I do, and we'll just see what happens."

Laura: It just really surprised me that I reacted that way, because I've always gotten hurt easily in the past. Things that shouldn't have bothered me so much really bothered me, so . . .

Dr. Sears: Yeah.

Laura: I thought, "Wow. Something's changed." And I didn't even tie it to this. But maybe it is related.

Dr. Sears: I do find that this course helps us with challenges at two general levels. One is being more present in the moment while it is happening. Noticing what comes up in the moment, and making a more conscious choice of how to respond. And then there's a more general self-care piece. We'll do this more consciously in the next few sessions. Planning how I can take care of myself better, which includes simple things like noticing I need to get more sleep, exercising regularly, and having more "down time." By doing things that bring my overall stress level down, I'm more tolerant when things do get difficult. I see those as two different, important pieces in dealing with stress. One is managing it as it's happening, and one is kind of inoculating yourself or reducing your general stress level. If the water level is up to your chin, every wave that comes along will be difficult to handle. But if the water level is only up to your knees, it's easier to handle the little waves that come by.

Kevin: I had one too, this week. It's actually a big one. While I haven't been able to work these last few weeks, I had an investment that was paying me several thousand dollars a month. It was carrying me during this time until I can get back working, but it stopped paying out. That was major. And it didn't bother me nearly as much as . . . it *should* have [laughter].

Dr. Sears: Well, now that you think about it . . . [laughter].

Stephanie: Well, I think it's bothering *me* a little bit [laughter].

Dr. Sears: Right, big things will always bother us, but with practice, they knock us off our feet less often. By accepting things as they are, even if they're difficult, we can make wiser choices.

Let me read a couple of things that give a sense of this theme of acceptance that we've been talking about. And again, this doesn't mean I have to like it when terrible things are happening. You may need to do something about the terrible things. But it starts with noticing things as they are. The first one is actually a poem by Rumi. Sometimes a poem can carry a sense of something, or an attitude or feeling, that is hard to describe. It's called *The Guest House*.

[Reads poem from MBCT protocol book]

Dr. Sears: For me, this conveys the sense of just being open to whatever comes along.

Stephanie: Yeah.

Dr. Sears: Especially when it's your own body, and your own thoughts, and your own feelings. It's funny how often we create a war with ourselves. We can practice showing ourselves some kindness and compassion, and letting these thoughts and feelings just be there.

The other one is a story about a king and his three sons.

[Reads story from MBCT book (Segal, Williams, & Teasdale, 2013) about a king who realizes he needs to learn to live with his unpopular son instead of spending all the energy and resources of his kingdom trying to keep him at a distance]

Stephanie: Wow!

Dr. Sears: So that's a powerful story. We spend a lot of time and energy trying not to feel bad feelings, or trying not to think thoughts we don't like, or trying not to feel uncomfortable. We are learning to meet our experiences as they are, and still move on, still have important things in our lives that we're moving toward.

Remember the attitude we're fostering is that important piece of "nonjudgmentally," or choosing to temporarily suspend our automatic judgments, which I know is challenging. Thoughts can easily creep in, like, "Gosh darn it, I'm thinking bad thoughts again!" or "Why can't I do better at this!" We can practice being kinder to ourselves, like, "Oh, isn't that interesting." I've even heard all of you saying that now. "Oh, isn't that interesting," "I just noticed that," and, "I got all upset about that, isn't that interesting." With this attitude, we're not fighting with ourselves all the time.

Kevin: I put in an order at my branch library for the *Full Catastrophe Living* book. It should be coming soon.

Dr. Sears: Oh, good. Any other comments while the projector is warming up for the video?

[Second half of *Healing From Within* video]

Dr. Sears: Any questions, comments?

Stephanie: It was amazing how the gentleman who had had so many back injuries, at the end, when they showed his face, there was not a wrinkle. His face just looked totally smooth. That was amazing.

Kevin: He wasn't worrying about the future in that moment.

Stephanie: Really cool.

Dr. Sears: Can you imagine breaking your back three times?

Kevin: Yeah, that's bad.

Christine: When they were showing him with his son, that reminded me, I have nieces and nephews, and they're all six and under. I love being around them, because they don't worry about tomorrow. They're so much in the moment, and it makes me feel that way when I'm with them. And nothing is that big of a deal to them. And it's the same idea. They're aware of themselves and their bodies. They tend to be self-centered, as naturally kids are. But I enjoy being with them, because they have those characteristics you just want to have yourself.

Dr. Sears: I agree. That's why I try to get across that mindfulness is a natural thing. It's not anything new, or magical, or hidden, or secret. It's just a natural way of being. But I think as we grow up, over time, we take on more and more life responsibilities, and we're tricked into thinking that we need to work hard for some great thing that's coming in the future. That's when we'll get our big reward. So we keep thinking of the next thing, and the next thing, and the next thing, and then before we know it, life is over. And we kind of miss the journey itself.

Stephanie: No kidding!

Dr. Sears: Anything else about the video?

Stephanie: I liked when Jon Kabat-Zinn said something about being aware of the little things.

Dr. Sears: Oh yeah, which Kevin brought up earlier, about the little things.

Stephanie: The little things are life.

Dr. Sears: Right. From a young age, it's just like, "Wait till you get to go to school! Won't that be great? And then you'll get to be in second grade. Then third grade!" On and on. There's always *something* you're waiting for, and then everything will be great. You miss so many of the moments you are in.

Christine: And then you want them back after they're over. It's not very helpful.

Dr. Sears: Who was it that said youth is wasted on the young? Yeah, just fostering that appreciation.

Stephanie: When my son was about 7 or 8, I think it was around Christmas, he made the comment, "I don't want to grow up. Being a kid is fun!" And I said, "Well, the good thing about that is by the time you get to be an adult, you'll be tired of being a kid." But when he said that, I thought, "I think I'm doing okay as a parent then if he likes being a kid."

Dr. Sears: Yeah, he's enjoying it—that's great.

Well, let's look at the home practice. Continue doing the sitting meditation this week. Every other day, try it without listening to the CD, just to see what happens. Everybody has different experiences. I've had some people say, "You know, sometimes I'm just really into it, and the CD annoys me by constantly talking." Other people say, "My mind drifts off too much, so I really like having the structure of the CD." So, just experiment and notice if there is a difference for you.

Stephanie: One of the things that I did do too on my phone is that I created a voice memo. And I have a little chime, and I chimed every minute.

Dr. Sears: Oh, that's interesting.

Laura: I was thinking about that too—how would I do the exercise without listening to the recording? I don't know that I would have a concept of each minute. That's a good idea.

Stephanie: It was funny, because it was 8 o'clock when I made my recording, and I could hear the clock ticking.

Laura: Where did you make the recordings you gave us? Because in a couple, I hear like a truck braking [laughter].

Kevin: I heard a bird [laughter].

Dr. Sears: That's funny, because in the last group, when I suggested they try listening to mindfulness recordings by other people, a couple of them said, "But I'm used to the way you do it, and at a certain time there's always the sound of a truck or of brakes." I made the recording in my office, and in the background every once in a while there's traffic. I tried to cut some of that out, but I was not in a professional studio with a soundproof room. Sorry about that [laughter].

Laura: That's great.

Kevin: I like those cues too. Like at one point, right before you come back in talking, I can hear you sort of [makes sound of licking lips] [laughter].

Dr. Sears: [laughter] You can hear me wet my whistle? Here comes my voice! Wow, I'll have to turn the volume down a little bit next time! [laughter]

Kevin: Hey, I'm paying attention to the sounds!

Stephanie: That's funny.

Dr. Sears: All right [laughter]. The other part is ideally to practice sitting with a difficulty at the end of the sitting meditation, even if only for five minutes or so. And then you might end with the three-minute breathing space to come back to the moment. It's a wonderful practice to be able to realize, "I can sit with difficult things, and they're not going to kill me." I can let it be here, whether or not it gets better. It may break up and dissipate, or it could be that you realize that you truly are angry about it. But it starts with noticing things as they are, and noticing how we tend to react. It can be a very interesting process to experiment with moving into things instead of pushing them away.

Stephanie: I like it.

Christine: What are your thoughts on using relaxing music very quietly in the background? Is that something that pulls you away from the exercise?

Dr. Sears: You know, a number of people ask that, and I think that's totally up to you. My suggestion is just to experiment. I'm sort of an amateur musician, and I like music, so when I hear it, I immediately go into it. So that would be distracting for me, because I'd be into it too much. For other people it sets the mood, and makes things easier.

Christine: I don't mean any great songs, just . . .

Dr. Sears: Oh, yeah, I know what you mean. Like some soft background music.

Christine: Like massage music.

Dr. Sears: Definitely experiment. I had one person say, "I like to just play it while I'm doing work around the house and dishes and things."

Stephanie: The meditations?

Dr. Sears: Yeah, the meditations. Actually, she had ADHD—attention problems. I told her that was okay, but my suggestion was to see if she could try just sitting with it too. She probably had a strong urge, "I gotta move!"

Kevin: It might help her to bring attention to whatever she's doing.

Dr. Sears: Exactly, yeah, as she's doing it. So, experimentation is good. But part of the course is to try things you might not have done if you were doing this on your own.

And the other two assignments are the same. Do the three-minute breathing space at regular times so you're not only doing it when you're stressed out. And then again, the hardest part is, like you said, when you're in the middle of the stress, can you somehow remember to move into it or breathe into it? The three minutes is a little bit arbitrary. If you don't have as much time, or you don't have a watch, it's really okay. You'll get a feel for it. It's about checking in with yourself, even if only for three breaths. Three minutes is good, because it doesn't feel like it's too overwhelming to do, yet gives time to get in touch with our experiences.

Stephanie: Good.

Dr. Sears: Any other comments or questions? And I'm five minutes over again. All right—see you again next week.

Laura: This is a class I don't mind going over.

Dr. Sears: Oh, well good! It's just that sometimes people have families waiting.

Stephanie: Thank you, Richard!

Dr. Sears: My pleasure.

10 Session 6

Thoughts Are Not Facts

Session six involves learning to relate differently to our thoughts. It is both obvious and profound to realize that thoughts and words represent reality but are distinctly different from reality. Recognizing this, instead of answering or arguing with our thoughts, we can pause to notice their patterns. We can see that strong negative thoughts are often symptoms of underlying emotions and moods. Instead of struggling with ruminative thoughts, we can see them as indications that we are becoming overwhelmed, and we can "decenter" from them. Instead of getting caught up in them, we can watch them, explore underlying body sensations, or take some considered action to take care of ourselves or the situation.

This session reviews more concepts from cognitive therapy, such as common patterns of maladaptive thinking, but emphasizes the importance of relating to them with curiosity and kindness.

In this session, I used Tibetan bells to provide sounds during the mindful listening part of the sitting meditation.

Session 6 Transcript

Dr. Sears: So, any burning questions or comments before we jump in with the exercise? All right, we're actually going to do the same one that we did last week, just practicing it some more.

[Sitting meditation—breath, body, sounds (ringing a bell), thoughts, difficulty]

Kevin: How long was that?
Dr. Sears: About 20 minutes, maybe longer.
Laura: Did it feel longer?
Kevin: It felt like a good 20, 25 minutes [laughter].
Dr. Sears: So what did people notice during that exercise? What came up?
Laura: I love that bell sound. I don't know why, I just like listening to it slowly fade out.
Dr. Sears: You know, I find that, too. It's like it really grabs my attention, and then as it gets quieter, it feels like my thoughts get quieter with it. I've always liked that, meditating with a bell.

Stephanie: I was aware of my third eye. It was like a lot of pressure. And I'm not sure why. Just a lot of pressure here at different times. And when you said, "Be aware of your thoughts," I was thinking about how I had an issue with my hip at one point, and I saw an acupuncturist. As he was going through and doing different points, as he was moving up my body, I could feel this pressure right here, and I mentioned it to him. And then he put a needle right there.
Laura: What did it feel like?
Stephanie: It hurt! And it's like, "Oh!" My thoughts kind of went to that. And I kept thinking, "No, it's not going to happen right now, it's all right." And it was a really small needle. It hurt just a little bit, but it was more of a shock than anything.
Laura: Did the acupuncture help?
Stephanie: I'm not sure. My hip is better. But I mean, it wasn't better at the time, so I don't know. I think stretching and doing some yoga helped. And walking every day.
Dr. Sears: You said you noticed the pressure today at different times. Did you notice any correlation between what you were thinking or feeling and when you noticed it more or less?
Stephanie: Just when we were doing the breath exercise.
Kevin: When you rang the bells, I could actually visualize the sound, like, in space. And it felt like when you first rang it, when it's at its

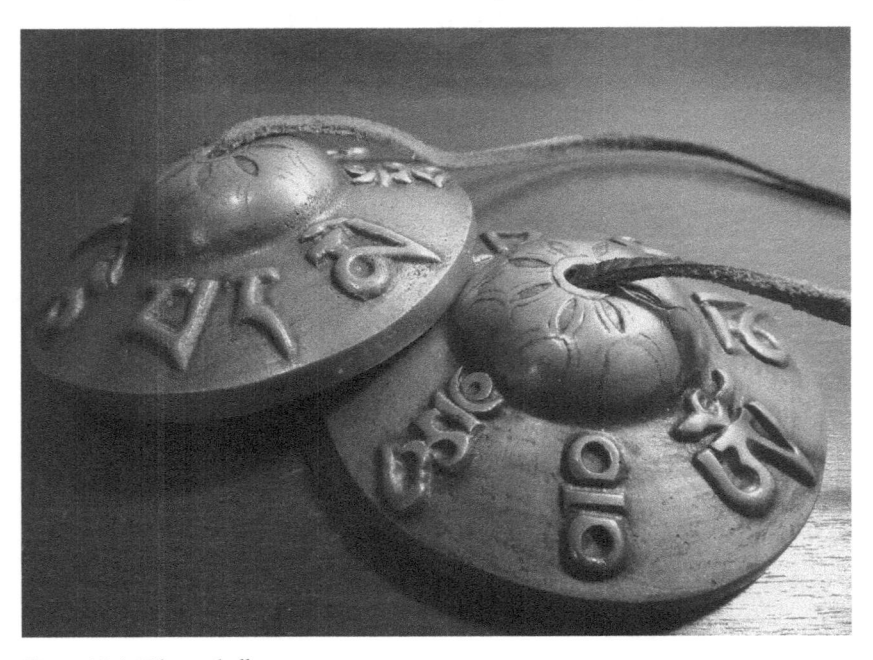

Figure 10.1 Tibetan bells

loudest, it's sort of up here, and as it eased, it came back towards the source itself. Physically, that's how it felt.

Dr. Sears: So you noticed images and feelings as you listened. I noticed an image of ripples in my mind as I heard the variety of overtones and oscillations.

Stephanie: They were loud—I'm glad you warned us. Because I've heard bells like that before, but not quite that sharp.

Dr. Sears: Yeah, they are designed more to wake up and stimulate, rather than relax you like a big bowl gong.

Kevin: Plus, you struck them skillfully [laughter].

Dr. Sears: How about working with the difficulty? How was that going? That's really one of the biggest lessons of this course—noticing and sometimes choosing to sit with something difficult. Even though it's not pleasant, and it doesn't go away, can you get more comfortable staying with it?

Laura: Just then, I couldn't seem to focus on any one. The past few days, there hasn't been anything hugely negative. So I thought, "Okay, maybe this would be appropriate to think about." But then I realized, "Well, that turned out okay."

Dr. Sears: Interesting. So that's a good experience by itself. We often push down things that bother us, but to have the ability to say, "Oh, you know, that wasn't so bad," and to be able to stay with things longer, can help us shift how we relate to difficulties.

Laura: Well, the specific thing I was thinking about, was that yesterday I had run a half-marathon for the first time. I've never run more than a 10K. So I'd went with a bunch of friends, and there were a few of us that were like, "Oh, we're gonna walk part of it," and "Oh, I'll run six or seven miles." When I got to mile seven, I thought, "Why don't I keep going?" And by mile eight I was in a lot of pain. But I didn't quit, I just kept going. And that's what I was thinking about, the pain that I was feeling at that time. I don't know if this class helped with it or not. Like, "Okay, I'm feeling this pain, but I'm not going to let it stop me, I'll just be aware of it."

Dr. Sears: It's about conscious choice. You might decide, "Yeah, this isn't worth it, seven is pretty good." But it sounds like you made a very conscious choice. Not, "I've got to quit," or "I've got to go on." You thought, "Yeah, I feel it, and I think I'll just keep going."

Laura: Yeah, and at one point I was thinking, "Is this pain okay to push through? Or is this pain telling me to stop?"

Stephanie: That's really cool!

Kevin: You ran 13 miles?

Laura: Yeah, I ran the whole time. I couldn't believe I did it. This is so ridiculous, but when I go and do stuff like this, I think, "If I finish this, I can post on Facebook that I ran the whole thing, and then everybody is going to say 'how wonderful!'" [laughter]. And

	I thought about that when I was running. My Facebook friends must be tired of it, but I get so many people that say, "Wow, that's great!" It's such great motivation. It was so much fun. Hundreds of people came out to cheer on the runners. 18,000 people ran. 11,000 ran the half, and 7,000 ran the marathon. And for the first 13 miles, you're all running together, the half-marathoners and the marathoners. And then when we get to the finish line, they keep going and do another 13 miles. But there were people lined up almost the whole route, shouting encouragement, holding up signs.
Kevin:	That helps.
Laura:	It does! It totally does. I think I would've quit if it hadn't been for that.
Stephanie:	I think I'll visualize that while I'm meditating! Going past the signs!
Laura:	When I first started running six months ago, I couldn't even run a half mile. So I would run, then I would walk. Then, by the time I was up to two or three miles, I started visualizing people cheering me on as I was running. Yes, it was great that it actually happened! And it was so awesome. There were signs that said "Way to go, complete stranger!" and I thought, "Yeah, that's for me!" [laughter]. It was a good experience. Sorry if I kind of went off on a tangent there!
Dr. Sears:	No, it really fits in with noticing and conscious choice, which we can apply to so many things in our lives. I decided I wanted to do this, and there's going to be obstacles and pain, and I can decide if I will stay with it or not.
Stephanie:	And while you're running and being in the moment, and seeing the sign that said "Way to go, complete stranger!" that was so cool!
Laura:	I wore a pink outfit and bunny ears, and I even pinned a little bunny tail on the back. [laughter] I asked a friend of mine who was going with me, "Should I do this?" and they're like, "Oh yeah, there's gonna be a lot of people in costumes." There was almost nobody in costumes! [laughter] It was great, because we were walking to where we line up for the race, and I'm like, "I'm still not seeing any costumes here!" But it turned out to be great, because people would yell things specifically at me, like, "Go, rabbit, go!"
Kevin:	Run, rabbit, run!
Laura:	And there were some cute little kids that would stand on the side and reach out their hands to give a high-five.
Kevin:	You're a star!
Laura:	I know, I feel like it! It's like every race I run now, I'm gonna do something!
Dr. Sears:	Awesome. Well it's hard to top that! What experiences did others have today sitting with a difficulty?
Stephanie:	I actually put an offer in on a house about a month ago, and I was a back-up bidder. They kept saying, "We don't think these people

will be able to pull this off." I found out Friday or Saturday that they had closed, so I didn't get the house. And so now I'm looking for a house, and there's a part of me that trusts the process, but there's a part of me that really wanted that house! It was just the right price, and it was just a lot of what I wanted.

Laura: That must've been very disappointing.

Stephanie: It was. I have a plan, and it's just not going according to my plan. So, whenever you had us focus on that, one of the things that I was aware of is that it will be all right. I will be okay. And I think it was shortly after that, when you asked us to become aware of our feelings and our emotions, that I was aware of that, "I'm okay. I'm content in this moment. I'm okay."

Dr. Sears: I was going to ask if you had that as a felt sense, because sometimes it is a thought saying, "It will be okay," but we don't really believe it—we're trying to convince ourselves. Then it's this weird conflict going on, versus noticing the feeling that's there, and the thoughts just kind of naturally rising.

Stephanie: And the emotions were—I was at peace. I've had emotions here, that's for sure! But it was peaceful.

Dr. Sears: Did it start off stressful and fall into that, or did you notice that you felt better about it than you thought?

Stephanie: I've had disappointment, and a little bit of concern, about finding something that I really like, because this is the first time in my life where I've ever bought a house that I get to pick exactly what I want! Because I've always adapted to what someone else wants, and this time I get to pick what I want, and that's kind of exciting! And so I'm going to get what I want.

Laura: It's kind of liberating, isn't it?

Stephanie: It is!

Laura: Doing just what you want to do.

Stephanie: Yes!

Dr. Sears: As I was doing this exercise today, I chose to work with the fatigue I am feeling. I've worked the last three weekends in a row. I found places where it was almost like I was fighting the tired, which is not very helpful, right? If you're tired and you're fighting it, then you're going to be more tired! So just realizing I can relax into feeling tired, without necessarily getting lost in it and falling asleep. So that's what I was going with, just kind of accepting, "You know, I'm just tired right now," and staying with that.

Anything else on that exercise before we talk about the week?

Kevin: Well, for me, the moment was just yesterday as I was jumping out of a plane.

Dr. Sears: Like, literally?

Kevin: No, I'm kidding [laughter]. You know, I find when you say on the recording, or just now on the exercise, to focus on sounds, my

	mind is more likely to wander. And when you say to focus on your thoughts, it's much easier to go still. I've noticed that several times.
Dr. Sears:	Okay. Yeah, it's important to notice, because there's no right or wrong with that. It's learning how our own minds work.
Kevin:	And I noticed the clock literally goes "tick, tock," it's not just "tock, tock." Why is that? Why does it make two different sounds?
Dr. Sears:	I'm not sure, unless it has one of those back-and-forth kind of things.
Kevin:	Maybe like a pendulum.
Dr. Sears:	Good. So how did the week go? One of the assignments was to try sometimes without the CD and see how that goes. And another assignment was to remember during the day to do the three-minute exercise.
Kevin:	I can't go without the CD yet.
Dr. Sears:	Ok, well, it's good to know.
Stephanie:	I tried it without the CD a few times, and I could only go about seven minutes, and then I'm like, "Bing!"
Kevin:	Yeah, because I haven't yet internalized the timing of each phase. So if I do it by myself, I won't know, like, "Okay, for about five minutes, focus on this, and the next five with the sound."
Laura:	Were we supposed to do the longer one without the CD, or the three-minute one?
Dr. Sears:	Either, or both. The idea is just to experiment with it, to notice how it works for you. And you know, for the sake of the recording, I try to make it about the same, but for your practice, you may decide, "Well the sound thing is going great for me," and you just end it there. Or you get so in the moment right away that you kind of fly though your breath and the body, and go right to your thoughts, spending a lot more time on that. Or you bring up a difficulty that's more difficult than you thought it would be, so you stay with it longer. So in a sense, it can be a good thing to not be structured. Over time, you kind of develop cues, like I notice my legs starting to tingle after 20 minutes of sitting cross-legged. It's also good to put a clock or timer near you, so you don't have to worry about losing all track of time.
Kevin:	The three-minute one I can do without the recording.
Dr. Sears:	Any experiences with being at work, or noticing something going on, and remembering, "Oh, I can check in with myself right now." Sounds like you did it during your marathon.
Laura:	I do that at work, never three minutes at a time, but it helps. One of my stresses at work is I hate running behind. I hate having people waiting when patient flow gets disrupted and things aren't scheduled just right. In the past, I ended up getting completely stressed out by it, but now I just take a moment, breathe, and look at what my thoughts are about it. People don't get upset about

Session 6: Thoughts Are Not Facts 151

	waiting 15 minutes. They'd be upset if they had to wait an hour, but that never happens, so I shouldn't stress about it.
Dr. Sears:	That's important, because your thoughts are trying to help, thinking, "Wow, I need to do something!" But when you're in a situation where you can't run away, or you can't really do anything, then you can practice accepting, "Well, I can't do anything right now." Otherwise, our minds run off with, "Oh, gosh, if this one patient is behind now, then they're all going to be behind." So in your mind, you're already upsetting 20 people.
Laura:	So I've kind of changed the way I think about that. Not doing a concrete three minutes' time, but just noticing my reactions.
Dr. Sears:	Yeah. The goal is to integrate this into your life, not to add more stuff, so the three-minute one is designed to give people some kind of structure to start with, but once you get the feel of it, whatever works best for you is great.
Kevin:	Yeah, I mean, at the beginning of the recording, you even say it can be condensed into three breaths or one breath. During the week, I did try doing it when my anxiety was bad. It's a matter of degree for me. When it's really, really strong, it's too strong for those meditations to slow down or to calm down, and sometimes it's too much.
Laura:	Did your issues with anxiety build up gradually, or did all of a sudden you just start having a lot of anxiety?
Kevin:	It's not issue based for me, it's physiologically based. It emerged when I stopped using my medication, because I've been using it for many years. So an effect of stopping that, that's when it emerged.
Laura:	So it started suddenly after you stopped your medication? I'm just curious.
Kevin:	Not suddenly, but alarmingly. I can't recall if it came from that, or gradually built. I'm not really sure.
Dr. Sears:	And the trap that we can get into is, here's this physiological feeling which is very real, and then, as you said, "alarmingly," now our reaction to it is, "I don't like this!" And the reaction kind of gets us stuck in there. I get what you were saying, sometimes it feels overwhelming, and you're just trying to get through that moment. Something I would suggest is to just check in with yourself, and not necessarily try to make it go away in that moment. Just noticing, "Oh, this is really strong right now." That's mindfulness. It's not that it goes away, or that now I feel good, or now I'm happy. It's noticing, "Very strong feelings are here, and thoughts of being overwhelmed are here," and then choosing whether to go into them, or take a walk, or talk to your doctor about it, or whatever you decide to do. That's mindfulness. You're just bringing your attention to it and deciding consciously, instead of automatically reacting to it.

Kevin: Some unpleasant sensations actually do ease when you allow them to just be, and this one depends on the degree.

Dr. Sears: Mmm-hmm.

Stephanie: I've just been taking deep breaths, like 3 or 4 or 5 or 6 or 7, anytime I've been feeling overwhelmed. It may not be three minutes, but it might be a minute, and it helps get me grounded and just a little more focused. And it feels good.

Dr. Sears: Good. And again, I find even if in that moment it doesn't do much good, often you're preventing yourself from building up tension and reactions that might have made it worse.

Laura: Yesterday morning, we all stayed in a hotel, and then we drove to the races at 5:30 in the morning. When we got there, we got parked, and we're sitting in the car, and we're looking at the guy who drove us, and he said, "Well, I just want to rest here for 15 minutes." This other friend and I were like, "Well, we want to go to where we're supposed to be!" We were getting all stressed out. And one guy that came with us wasn't running, he was just there to take pictures and cheer us on. And so I'm sitting in the back and just realizing what I was doing, and he goes, "Just keep breathing." And I said "Oh! I'm sorry," and he said, "Just keep breathing." We all had to stop and take a few breaths.

Dr. Sears: That's funny, because it can start to have that ripple effect in people you know once they see it's working for you. All right, anything else about the week?

The theme for today is, "Thoughts are not facts," and the subtitle is, "even the ones that tell you they are." Let's start off with a scenario (Segal, Williams, & Teasdale, 2013). Imagine that you're feeling down because you've just had a quarrel with a colleague at work. Shortly afterward, you see another colleague in the general office, and he or she rushes off quickly, saying he or she couldn't stop. So just throw out what kind of thoughts pop into your mind after that kind of scenario.

Stephanie: She's going to avoid me forever!

Laura: So you had a quarrel with one person, and another person says, "Oh, I can't stop"?

Dr. Sears: Yes.

Stephanie: Another colleague? Yeah, they've already heard, that's what I'm thinking!

Laura: So the person I was talking to went and talked to them, so now that person doesn't want to talk to me.

Kevin: I didn't want to talk to them anyway.

Dr. Sears: Yeah, we might have all kinds of thoughts. So now imagine this scenario (Segal, Williams, & Teasdale, 2013). You're feeling happy, because you and a work colleague have just been praised for good work. Shortly after, you see another colleague in the general

	office, and he or she rushes off quickly saying he or she couldn't stop. What thoughts might come up?
Kevin:	They might feel like they're not good enough.
Laura:	You got praised, but he or she didn't.
Dr. Sears:	Jealousy, yeah. Interesting that you both went to the negative, because it could've been, "I guess they were busy!" It's funny where our minds tend to go. As we talked about before, our thoughts and our feelings are very connected. So if you have the thought, "Oh, they heard that we had an argument," or "they're jealous," that's going to have a certain impact on how you're feeling, as compared to thoughts like, "Oh, I hope they're okay," or "Oh, they must be having a busy day. I'll buy them a donut later." You'll have different feelings depending on the thoughts. Likewise, the mood you are in will influence the thoughts you have.

So what we want to practice doing is just noticing these thoughts as they come up. Normally, they're almost automatic, because they're in the background somewhere. We don't check them out, we just assume, "if it's a thought, it must be true." It may sound odd at first, yet it should also be obvious that a thought is a phenomenon that is separate from the reality it represents. Thinking about "water" is different than the experience of this liquid stuff here. Our thoughts represent reality, but they are not the same thing as the reality, so they may or may not match up.

So, we can develop the ability to recognize, "Oh, I'm noticing that I'm thinking this," and then it's up to me to decide if it's true or not. Have you ever had someone make an assumption about what you meant by something, and then an argument follows, but it was based on something that was not even true? Once a thought gets planted, a feeling can follow, and that affects the way you treat the other person, and then you kind of have this cascade. Even for thoughts about ourselves, like, "I'm no good," it sets off a chain of thoughts like, "Because I'm no good, then nobody is going to want to be around me, and if nobody wants to be around me, then I'm going to be lonely forever, and if I'm lonely my whole life, I'm going to die at a young age, and I'll have no kids . . ." So one thought about being no good gets you feeling that your entire life will be worthless. We all tend to do that, though hopefully not to that extreme all the time.

So we can learn to recognize, "Wow, I'm having a lot of catastrophizing thoughts right now—it must mean I'm stressed out." That's a whole different way to relate to your thoughts—seeing your thoughts as a barometer with information on how you're feeling. Instead of getting caught up in arguments with ourselves, like, "No, I am worthy!" "No, you're not!" "Yes, I am!", we can step back and notice, "Oh, wow, I'm arguing with myself about whether or not I'm a worthwhile person. That probably means I'm getting depressed. What are some things I can do to take care of myself now that I know I'm feeling overwhelmed?"

Of course, you may decide, "Actually, this thought is really important. What do I want to do with the rest of my life?" Maybe you went through some life change, and now you're not happy with your job. By noticing and sitting with it, you can decide if that is an important question, or if it is stemming from anxiety. That's a whole different thing than automatically getting worked up, as somebody who jumps around and tries different things and is never happy with anything. We're just learning to be more conscious of what we're doing.

So let me pass out the handouts for today. You can read through this on your own, but I'll point out a couple of things. The middle paragraph talks about how we can start to notice what thoughts are there, the patterns we have, and the "top ten" automatic thoughts we get when we're stressed. The more you're able to watch them, the less power they have over you. Like the first time you watch a horror movie, it's very scary. But if you've watched it 40 times, then you say, "Oh, yeah, this is the part where his head gets chopped off," and it's no big deal. Likewise, we can notice, "Oh, yeah, here's the part where I think I'm a loser again. I think that every time I have to give a presentation, because I'm worried people are going to judge me." You can learn that thoughts don't have to have such power over you, even when you may not be able to stop them. In fact, there have actually been studies that show if you try to stop your thoughts, you make them worse. Very often, strong thoughts are really coming out because you're stressed or overwhelmed, and the thoughts are trying to fix the stress.

Stephanie: Trying to protect you or warn you.

Dr. Sears: Yeah, because our thinking fixes things, so we think we can fix everything with our thinking, so we just keep going and going with thinking. By noticing the pattern, I can check in with my emotions and body sensations, I can choose to focus on what I'm doing in the moment again, or I can choose to do something to take care of myself. Doing this often robs the thoughts of their fuel, and they may just dissolve.

Kevin: I'm just—yeah, it is interesting. Trying to be aware of identifying thinking patterns and note them down.

Dr. Sears: It can be challenging, because we are usually "in" our thoughts, as part of the scene. It takes practice to step back and notice them. The next page of the handout talks about ways you can see your thoughts differently, so you have some options once you're aware of what these thoughts are. Maybe you recognize it's old stuff,

	like when I was working with someone who had been in a bad relationship for years. She would think about it constantly, like "Maybe if I think about it enough, I'll fix it, or I'll come up with the right thing to make him understand." She said she was cleaning out some emails, and found some from seven years ago that she had sent him, and was stunned to see that they were exactly the same thoughts she was still having about the relationship.
Laura:	The same person? She'd been with somebody that long, and was having the same thoughts about the same person seven years later?
Dr. Sears:	Yeah, the same kinds of things she constantly thought about, like how he was not emotionally available, how she was not a priority to him, and how he didn't keep his promises.
Stephanie:	I've done the same thing, though! That's why I'm thinking, "Of course!" That's amazing.
Dr. Sears:	Yeah, so developing that awareness of, "Wow, these thoughts keep coming up. Is this helpful or not?" It was a breakthrough for her to see that all these thoughts were just distracting her from the reality that she was in a bad relationship. She was choosing to suffer a smoldering dissatisfaction instead of feeling the awful grief of breaking up with him.

So, when thoughts come up and you can't get them out of your mind, here are some different things you can do with them. One is, as we're practicing, just watch them. Just let them come and go, without feeling like you have to follow them. Because again, we sometimes compulsively get caught up in them, like, "What if people don't like me?" "Oh, I'll make them like me by doing such and such." It's like we have to answer them all. We can realize, "Oh, there goes that thought that people don't like me. That often comes up when I get stressed." I don't have to fight it or answer it. I don't have to fix that thought before it'll go away. It just comes and goes by itself, as you may have started to notice in your practice. In fact, if you can't stop thinking about something, instead of trying to push it away, you can just decide to make it the focus of your awareness. You will often find it is hard to stay focused on it—the mind often drifts all over the place. So you could just sit there and watch it, "Okay, here's that thought, I'm just going to sit here and watch it, and notice what happens." Just like with pain, anxiety, and other difficulties we've practiced with, thoughts will also tend to break up and change when we move into them.

The next suggestion is to view your thought as a mental event rather than a fact. It may be true that this event often occurs with other feelings, and it is tempting to think of it as true, but it's up to you to decide if this thought is true or not, and how you want to deal with it.

	You can also write your thoughts down on paper. One of the reasons journaling is so helpful is because when your thoughts are on paper, you can more easily recognize that they are separate from you. You get a little distance and a little perspective.
Stephanie:	I noticed that when I write things down, I think, "That's what I've been focusing on? That's ridiculous!"
Dr. Sears:	Yeah, right. And again, it helps you see that your emotions at the time played a big part in the thoughts that were there.
Laura:	Sometimes I'll send emails to myself like I'm writing it to another person, but I don't send it to them. Like if I'm dating someone, and something's not going well, and I'm upset, I'll write them an email, send it to me, and then I reread it. . .
Stephanie:	I do the same thing!
Dr. Sears:	That's a great idea.
Stephanie:	Not to people I'm dating!
Dr. Sears:	You just have to watch the "To:" line very carefully so you don't accidentally send it to somebody!
Laura:	Sometimes to friends, or someone I had a conflict with, or something like that, I'll write it all out, and I just don't send it to them, but it helps me get those thoughts out.
Dr. Sears:	Right.
Stephanie:	And I have a little thing in my email, emails to myself . . .
Dr. Sears:	"You're beautiful, you're wonderful. . ."
Stephanie:	No, actually they're not! Usually it's a resentment or something like that I'm working on. I read it out, and it kind of helps me to see it.
Dr. Sears:	That's a great idea. Not to mention, if you do decide to send it, you can notice, "What would it look like if I got this email?

The fourth suggestion is to ask yourself questions about the thoughts that are popping up. So, did this thought just pop into my head automatically? Does it fit with the facts of the situation? Is there something about this thought I could question? How would I have thought about this at another time, in another mood? And are there alternatives? It could be you're dead on with the thought, but we can practice asking, "Could I think about this in a different way?"

The fifth one, for really difficult thoughts, is that it might be helpful to literally meditate on it, to just sit in meditation with it, noticing it with your "wise mind." I'm not sure if they're referring to the same thing, but in dialectical behavior therapy (Linehan, 1993), wise mind is the part of you that balances your rational mind and your emotional mind. Rational mind is that thinking, logical part of us, and we also have an emotional mind that takes our feelings about something as important. We can get stuck in one or the other, or sort of lean towards one or the other, but there is a wise mind in between that takes both into account. So this may be a super logical decision, but my heart tells me something else. When we sit with something, and get past the initial struggle and resistance, we can get more in touch with that balanced, wise place inside of us.

On the next page are suggestions from cognitive therapy, where we specifically are taught to work with our own thoughts. What you see in the last sentence is crucial. "The keynote attitude to take with your thoughts is gentle interest and curiosity" (Segal, Williams, & Teasdale, 2013, p. 323). Hopefully, you're beginning to understand what that means, because it sounds kind of funny if you haven't practiced the mindfulness exercises. "Oh, isn't that interesting, I keep thinking about choking my boss right now" [laughter]. Whether you use humor, or just kind of step back, the idea is to explore what is going on. It's also about learning to be kind to yourself. "Oh, this is curious, I can't stop thinking about this. I wonder what's going on right now, and how I'm feeling in my body." Just taking a gentler approach to your own experiences, even when they are difficult.

Stephanie: Those are good ones.

Dr. Sears: Yeah. "Am I confusing a thought with a fact?" "Am I jumping to conclusions?" "Am I thinking in black-and-white, meaning all-or-nothing, terms?" For the very same person, we may think, "Oh, they're wonderful, they're such a blessing," and then, "Oh, I hate their guts!" It's the same person, even if the behaviors change over time.

Stephanie: Drive me nuts!

Dr. Sears: "You're the best therapist I've ever had." "You're the worst therapist I've ever had." [laughter]

Stephanie: Have you heard that from the same person?

Dr. Sears: Probably, though I'd like to think not that often!

"Am I condemning myself totally because of one thing?" And again, some of these go along with depression. It's just how your mind starts to work in depression, like, "I messed up this one thing, but I feel like I messed everything up. I can't do anything right. Nobody's ever going to love me." This string of feelings and thoughts start to pop up, so we can begin to question those thoughts. "Concentrating on my weaknesses and forgetting my strengths." "Blaming myself for something that isn't my fault." Sadly, you especially see this in the extreme, like with abuse victims. "If I would've been nicer, they wouldn't have hit me." No, nobody deserves to be hit for any reason whatsoever. But we also blame ourselves in more subtle ways. "If only I'd have gone a different way in traffic, the accident wouldn't have happened." Well, how would you have known to go a different way in traffic?

"Am I judging myself?" "Am I setting unrealistically high standards for myself?" "Am I mind reading?" My wife does this all the time—she says she knows what I'm thinking, and then gets mad at me for it. I never do that [laughter]. There's also "crystal ball gazing," where you think you can predict the future, and you spend a lot of time worrying about "what ifs" that are not even likely to happen. "Am I expecting perfection?" And again, breaking out of these patterns of thinking begins with just recognizing them.

So the next couple of pages are just some things to think about. Kind of funny language—some thoughts to think about thoughts [laughter]. One of these tells a story about a guy who took the thoughts he put down on his to-do list very seriously. He had "wash car" on his list, so he found himself at ten o'clock at night turning on his floodlights in the yard and washing the car. He suddenly stopped and asked himself, "What the hell am I doing? Just because it was on my list, and I had a thought that I had to wash the car, doesn't mean it *has* to be washed! I can choose to do this another day!" But, you know, we all get caught up in our thoughts sometimes, as if they are the absolute truth, and we have to follow them.

Stephanie: I did that once, but it was . . .
Laura: You washed your car at ten o'clock at night?
Stephanie: No, I decided to wash my car, but it was 22 degrees. I went to a car wash, and I got the hose thing going, and all of a sudden it just froze onto my car! And I was like, "Why did I do that?" I didn't even think it all the way through.
Kevin: Yeah, this might not be the best time!
Stephanie: The soap was literally freezing onto my car. People must have been driving by like, "What is she doing?! Crazy woman!"
Dr. Sears: But *that* was just a thought! [laughter]
Stephanie: I give it a second thought now when I wash my car.
Dr. Sears: So, any questions or comments about anything? I really like the way this course is set up and how it progresses. In the meditation traditions I was first trained in, we didn't talk about things this explicitly. Maybe after a few years, you might get good enough to see your own thoughts clearly. For me, it's just so helpful to start with the body sensations, and then things like sounds, then to be able to recognize your thoughts, and then to learn how to work with difficult thoughts and feelings. For traditions that espoused celibacy and poverty, the practice might be, "Okay, now I'm noticing I'm thinking, and now I'm going to just breathe." Not to put that down, and they weren't all like that, but most of us also need to work in the daily world, and interact with people, and have relationships, and we can use that quality of attention

	to work with our thoughts and feelings, too. Most people really identify with the content of their thoughts. It's a big paradigm shift to say, "I *have* thoughts, I *have* feelings, I *have* sensations, but I'm much bigger than that. I'm the context of all of this."
Stephanie:	One thing I like about this program is discovering my mind is always going, and when I focus on my thoughts, I give them my attention, I can just let them swirl in my head. But also, that right here, right now, my thoughts are part of who I think I am, and so it's a way to challenge it. So I like it.
Dr. Sears:	Yeah, now that's a good way to say it's part of you right now. It's not a definition, or all that you are.
Stephanie:	No, and it gives me a chance to challenge those thoughts. That's great.
Dr. Sears:	Many of us almost live entirely in our heads, and spend so much time in our thinking that we're missing out on life and our experiences. As James Joyce said about one of his characters, "Mr. Duffy lived a short distance from his body."
Kevin:	My intuition tells me this is kind of a big leap this week—this is important.
Dr. Sears:	Yeah, and I think it's logical, and it makes sense intellectually, but it took us six weeks of practicing to be able to have some experience of it. As I've said, I don't have some sort of secret that you have to buy into or believe me on. Just practice for yourself, and notice what happens, and discover how it works for you. If from day one, I really tried to get across this material about thoughts, it would probably have seemed confusing, or too abstract and subtle. It actually takes some time to train your attention to be able to get to this capacity for noticing.

So anything else about today before we go into homework? |
| *Kevin:* | Yeah, this is a lot this week. |
| *Dr. Sears:* | Yeah, so I definitely recommend reading over the handouts several more times. So the home practice is to continue with the sitting meditation—breath, body, sounds, thoughts, and ideally, sitting with a difficulty. Also, start thinking about how you might customize your personal practice when the group is over. So think about, out of all the exercises we've done, which ones you connect with the most, the best times of day to do them, and consider a regular practice that you might look forward to and enjoy doing for self-care, as opposed to, "Oh, I have to do this all the time."

Well, there are only two more classes, so make sure you ask all the questions you need to. Of course, everyone can contact me after the course is over, and I've been planning to start some kind of continuing "refresher" classes, maybe monthly, where people can reconnect with the practice. |
| *Laura:* | I think that would be helpful. |

Dr. Sears: I think so, too.
Laura: When I'm doing something like this, when I'm doing a class, I'm pretty good with keeping up with it, and then when it ends, I go back to my old habits.
Dr. Sears: That's a really good point. We'll talk a lot more about keeping up the momentum in the last session.

The other two assignments are to continue with the breathing space, practicing it regularly and remembering to do it when you begin to feel stressed.

All right, any other questions? Comments? Complaints?
Stephanie: See where your mind is.
Laura: This has been a good class.
Dr. Sears: Oh, good. All right, we'll see you next week.

11 Session 7
Taking Care of Myself

In this session, we emphasize the importance of noticing as the first step in dealing with challenges. When things begin to get bad, we often fall into old patterns, such as ignoring the situation or pretending it is not really happening and hoping it will go away. By learning to pay attention to the signs of oncoming stress, anxiety, or depression, we can take proactive steps to take care of ourselves before we get too overwhelmed.

It is difficult to dig your way out of a deep hole, but if you notice you are just starting to slide down into one, it can be easier to climb back up. It is even better to notice the holes before you fall into them. This session is about noticing the factors that lead to becoming overwhelmed, our unique "relapse signatures." By creating our own personal plan ahead of time, we are better prepared to take preventive action, knowing that our thoughts and feelings will follow later.

Session 7 Transcript

Dr. Sears: So we made it to session seven! That is really a big accomplishment by itself.

Laura: Why, do some people not?

Dr. Sears: Actually, most of them do. But it's a big commitment to stick with it and come here eight times. Often in the first few weeks, thoughts come up like, "I don't know if I'm getting this," or "This is a lot more work than I thought it might be." So just setting this time aside for your own self-care is a pretty big deal. Of course, we also ask everyone to pay up front as encouragement to keep coming [laughter]. All right, any burning questions or comments before we jump into the exercise?

Kevin: I started writing down my top 10 negative and positive thinking patterns. I've got 8 negatives and 4 positives so far.

Dr. Sears: Good! And you're noticing our brain's tendency to more easily notice the negative.

All right, this is going to be the same set of exercises we did last week.

[Sitting meditation—breath, body, sounds (with bells), thoughts, difficulty]

Dr. Sears: And before we end, I would just like to read a poem to you, so just listen and see if it evokes anything for you. It's called "The Summer Day," by Mary Oliver. [Reads poem]

So what did people notice? What did you experience?

Christine: What is the deal with the bells? What exactly are they for? I know they are on a couple of the other sections of the CD. If I don't turn it off, they go on to the next one. I've heard them before.

Dr. Sears: These are Tibetan ones, specifically. We talked about them last week—these give more of a waking up, jolting sound. You've probably seen the big bowl ones that give more of a mellow, relaxing, "bong" sound.

Christine: And it is just to bring your attention back?

Dr. Sears: Yes, it is just one more way of engaging the senses, just like incense for smell, or body movement for touch. Traditionally, when you had a room full of people, instead of shouting, "Hey, everybody, let's start meditating," you would have codes. In some traditions, you hear three bells to signal the start of the meditation, and one signals the end. When you are sitting all day long, your legs will go to sleep, so what they typically do is put a walking meditation in between the sitting ones. So every 20 or 30 minutes, or sometimes every hour depending on how sadistic the leader is [laughter], they will ring the bell so everybody knows when it is time to stand up and walk around.

For me, the sound of the bells fills my mind, and as the sound fades, it feels like my mind is getting quieter, as my thoughts are kind of fading with it. It's just one more thing you can use as a meditation tool. Over time, you can even condition your body to trigger a relaxation response, because the sound gets associated with being in the moment. You can even put a program on your phone called "Mindfulness Bell," which you can set to go off hourly or randomly with a soft "ding," which reminds you to drop into the moment more often throughout the day.

What else did people notice or experience?

Laura: So when we're supposed to concentrate on some difficulty, it's really hard not to try to figure out a solution to it. That's challenging.

Dr. Sears: It's important to notice that tendency. You know, we're not saying never try to figure out a solution—sometimes we need to. But when we get stuck just constantly thinking about stuff, we can also choose to sit with it, and let go of the compulsion to constantly try to figure it out, which often ends up being a subtle way of avoiding the feeling it brings up in our bodies.

Much like with physical pain, if you are tightening up against a difficulty, you can learn to notice that, and you can begin to let go of some of the tension and resistance around it.

I even find that instead of fighting with it, if I let it sit there, if there is a solution, it will sometimes come by itself. After all, you can't force yourself to think harder. Muscle tension doesn't help. I also think it's important, especially with this inner work, to know that it doesn't always feel like it gets easier when you sit with something difficult. It could just be that you become more aware of the layers and the subtleties that you weren't aware of before, or you're just more overwhelmed than you thought you were. The goal is to begin with noticing more, not necessarily always making it fun and easy.

Laura: I thought that was the goal, to make it fun! [laughter]

Dr. Sears: Interestingly, the side effect is that it becomes more fun and easy over time, because you learn to let go of struggling with yourself. But you can fall into this trap, where the more you are trying to become happy, and constantly comparing this moment to what happiness should feel like, the more you are fighting and not experiencing the moment as it is, and the more you are really going to end up pushing it away. In fact, there's a book called *The Happiness Trap* (Harris, 2008). By letting go of trying to be happy, and just flowing more fully with your experiences moment by moment, the more likely you'll be happy. It's one of those paradoxes.

Kevin: Well, I definitely couldn't solve or control the situation that I brought up during the difficult situation, because I was reflecting on the weather. Definitely couldn't do much about the weather. At least four consecutive days of no sunshine.

Laura: Are you affected quite a bit by that?

Kevin: Oh, yeah.

Dr. Sears: Well, normally, we might react with, "Dang, I wish it'd hurry up!", or "It's not fair!", or "Why does this keep happening?!" But if you get stuck in that all the time, it's just wasted energy and effort. It doesn't change the weather. So just noticing, "Oh, yeah, I'm reacting again. I need to just sit with this, and decide what I want to do, if anything." Your feeling of frustration may just pass, or you might decide to fly to Florida.

All right, anything else on this exercise today before we talk about the week? How about awareness of thoughts? How's that coming along, because I think it's a pretty subtle thing to notice what our own thoughts are. I think there are layers, some that are loud and strong, and some that are sort of drifting around in the back of the mind.

Laura: It's not always easy to do that. Sometimes, I'll imagine myself writing them in a journal, to try and see them.

Dr. Sears: So you are practicing ways to notice them. And you were saying that you were making a list of your top negative and positive thoughts.

Kevin: Patterns, yeah, thought patterns. I think those would be good to know if I want to work with a coach or therapist after this class. Those would be good themes, like one per week or something. Looking at this particular tendency or thought pattern. Not spending too much time on why I might have it, but a little, maybe. And then trying to look at it from different angles, and looking at alternatives to it.

Dr. Sears: Yeah, well said, because I think sometimes we can go into too much "I've got to know exactly why I think this way and where it came from," and then we are more stuck, because we're trying to figure out the thinking with more thinking. I think it would be interesting to notice, "I'm wondering if this thinking pattern came from how I grew up." Of course, just knowing that is not always enough. It just gives you some leverage on it. And by stepping back, you can say, "Oh, well that's because my childhood stuff is coming up again." That's another way of getting that distance. Then you can decide what you want to do with it.

What else came up during the week? How about the three-minute exercise? Sounds like it's working for you, just a shortened version during the day?

Laura: I had a bad day today, and did that twice. The full three minutes. One of the employees quit. It's very stressful to find someone and get them trained. I thought, "I need to stop for a few minutes and not get overwhelmed by this."

Dr. Sears: I salute the fact that you decided to take care of yourself, because I think too often it's like, "Oh, this is so stressful, I've got to do something about it right away," and we tend to forget about our own well-being. We're going to talk more about that today, but just recognizing, "This is stressful, let me take care of myself, and then I'll be in a better place to deal with the problem."

Laura: Yeah, that's exactly what I was thinking. If I get all upset about this, it's not going to do me or anybody else any good.

Kevin: What field are you in?

Laura: I'm an optometrist.

Dr. Sears: Anything else about the week?

Christine: I tried listening to the sitting meditation with relaxing background music that is meant for meditating or massage or something. It seemed to help some. It calmed my brain down a bit more.

Laura: Where did you get it? What music did you use?

Christine: There are two that I use a lot. One's called Calm the Mind and the other one is Stress something-or-other. They aren't songs that

	you would recognize. It's just relaxing music, and to put that in the background of the sitting meditation helped me be able to stop thinking so much about everything.
Dr. Sears:	That's great.
Christine:	It made it more of a relaxation exercise.
Dr. Sears:	To me, it's good to experiment to find what helps. Music is another example of something that is happening right then and there, engaging our senses, and changing from moment to moment. Instead of going off in your thoughts, you're bringing it back to the sound of music. That's great.
Kevin:	I ended up, I kind of foreshadowed this was going to happen this week, because when you gave us the material last week I could tell that for me this was sort of the meat of the matter of the mindfulness. Identifying our negative thought patterns. And I found myself this week looking at those pages and reading those through several times, what you gave us, and I got away from the three minutes. I didn't do the three minutes and sitting meditation nearly as much as I had in previous weeks. It just kind of naturally, my attention just kind of shifted to the patterns.
Dr. Sears:	Sounds like you made a conscious choice to move into something that is important. The more you see these patterns as separate from you, the more you can sort of get leverage over them. If it feels like they're controlling you, you can notice, "I'm still having these thoughts, and I'm noticing these feelings are present, but I can decide what I can do about them, if anything."

Once you get this concept and experience of just being present, you can do it with anything. I've had people say that they mindfully crochet. Instead of talking and looking around everywhere, you can practice feeling it, noticing it, and letting your thoughts stay with what you are doing as a purposeful exercise. You can practice paying attention during any activity, whether building models, surfing, gardening, or taking a walk. The danger, I think, is that you can slip back into doing it in automatic pilot mode if you are not conscious. In other words, if you tell yourself, "I am not going to do meditation anymore. I am just going to make walking my meditation," you can start out with a good intention, but over time you are just walking automatically again and daydreaming the whole time. That's fine if you want to do that, but if you want to maintain your mindfulness muscles, it is important to get into the habit of consciously deciding, "This is my time to just be present."

All right, anything else before we talk about the themes for today?

If you have some paper, you can use that, otherwise, you can write on today's handout. This is just for you—you don't have to turn this in to anybody. What I want you to do is write down a list of activities you do on a daily basis. Now if every day is different for you, as you just told me, just pick a recent day. From the time you wake up until the time you go to bed, what activities do you do on a typical day? Just write down maybe fifteen or twenty for now, and you can go back and put in more detail later if you want. For now, what we want to do is get down on paper what you do throughout the day.

[pause]

You can keep working on that, but what I would like you to do next is go back through your list, and put an "N" next to the activities in your day that are nourishing or nurturing, in other words, that give you energy or bring you up. And put a "D" next to the activities that are draining or depleting, the ones that take away energy or bring you down.

Christine: What if they're neutral? Just leave them?

Dr. Sears: Yeah, some may be neutral. Sometimes people also tell me that the same activity can be either one, depending on the day or the circumstances, so you can write "N/D."

[pause]

So again, you can go back and do this in more detail on your own later, but what did you notice as you did this exercise? Was there anything about your list that surprised you, or something that came up for you?

As you look at this, it is important to realize, THIS is your life. You know, we often live in our heads, or think that some "better" future is coming, but in a very real way, you are looking at the moments that constitute your life. It can be interesting to see it on paper.

Did people have more Ns, or more Ds, or is it balanced? What did people notice?

Laura: I have a lot of N/D.

Dr. Sears: Okay, so you have a lot of activities that are nourishing on some days and are draining on other days?

Laura: Yeah, a simple thing like taking a shower and getting ready. Sometimes, that is a good part of the day, and sometimes it's like, "Oh, shit, I haven't allowed enough time, I'm running late!" It's stressful. "I've got to get ready to go!"

Dr. Sears: Okay, so maybe time is one of the factors in that case that makes something an N or a D for you.

Laura: And, I think, I hate to use the word "addicted," because I think that's too strong of a word, but I'm a little bit addicted to checking Facebook and checking my e-mail. I look forward to doing that stuff, but it tends to just not be a nourishing activity. Usually, I get too obsessed with it, and it's a draining thing.

Dr. Sears: That's good to notice.

Laura:	Yeah, but I don't know how to stop doing that. Even though I know, when I sit there and do that for too long, that I don't feel good afterwards, I still do it. I don't know how to stop doing it.
Dr. Sears:	Well, we can talk more about that if you want to, but one step is now that you have more awareness, more mindfulness, you can ask, "What am I noticing about myself when I get the urge to check?" That typically will be some anxiety, or some loneliness, or maybe some sadness. It could even be excitement, "I'm curious to know what my friend has done last night." And then you can decide, "I'll check right now," or "I'm feeling all that, but I think I'll just wait a little bit longer before I check it." And then, you're inserting a conscious choice, and you can decide. You can practice waiting a little longer each time, or just check at certain times instead of constantly. You may even decide, "This is my guilty pleasure that I want to indulge in." But by noticing the urges, the feelings, and the judgments, what you choose to do will be more conscious and less driven.
Kevin:	This might not be an issue for you at all, but for me, since anxiety is a big challenge, sometimes I can't really bear to sit in front of the computer, but I can bear to check e-mail on my phone. There is a difference, because the computer is on a desk in a room, and the phone I can walk outside if I want and check e-mail. There's a big difference.
Dr. Sears:	So what did you notice?
Kevin:	Well, I'm not working these days, so I got almost all Ns.
Dr. Sears:	That's a nice place to be—sometimes we take it for granted when things are going well. It's also interesting how often people will say, "Oh my gosh, I have Ds all over the place. I didn't realize!" It's no wonder we are stressed or depressed or worn out when our whole day is filled with draining activities. So as you look at your list, consider, "Are there some activities I could just cut back on? Maybe I am doing it automatically, or because I thought I was expected to, and maybe I can do it less often, or reduce it, or shift it to somebody else." Some things you just have to do, even if you find them draining, like feeding your kids [laughter]. In those cases, are there any ways you can reduce how draining they are? I was working with somebody who said, "Whenever I know I've got to go into a tough meeting, I always make myself a nice cup of chamomile tea. It just gives me something to smell, something to taste, and it's just a little concrete thing I can hold on to knowing that I've got to deal with some difficult things." The other question is, how can you build into your day more nourishing activities? We can fall into this pattern of, "I've got to do this, I've got to do that, I've got to take care of everybody else," and usually, if there is time left over, we take care of ourselves. We

can more consciously ask, "Where can I insert more Ns into my day?" They don't always have to be huge things, like long vacations, just little things to help you take care of yourself.

Another thing that is important about nourishing activities is that they can be further divided into pleasurable and mastery activities. Things that are pleasurable are obviously nourishing. We don't always think of it this way, but an activity that gives us a sense of mastery can also be nourishing. In other words, whether or not we like the activity itself, when it's done, we feel good because we accomplished something.

Christine: Like when I'm in the city, running errands, like going to the grocery. I don't like to do that, but when it's done, I feel like I accomplished something, which then can be nourishing.

Dr. Sears: Right, exactly. So it's important to have both of those kinds of things. That becomes really important when we are feeling overwhelmed, especially with depression. Typically, if we don't feel like doing something, we say, "I don't feeling like doing that. I'm going to rest." Normally, that may be a good idea. But if your issue, especially, is depression, you need to do the opposite. You have to make yourself do it, and the feelings will catch up later, sometimes much later. If you decide to wait until you feel like it, you are going to withdraw from activities and people. The more you withdraw, the more depressed you get, because you aren't getting anything done, and then you get depressed about that. Your mood then continues to spiral downward.

Normally, we might find ourselves sometimes saying, "I'm just so tired, I don't want to be around people. I'm not going to go out tonight." And that's usually not a big deal, but in terms of depression, that can easily slip into the next night, then the next night, then the next night. Then you become isolated socially, and don't have any support from friends, and then you get more depressed about being lonely, and down goes your mood in a vicious spiral.

By practicing mindfulness, we can notice this pattern developing before we get overwhelmed, and then do something proactively to nurture ourselves. As a matter of fact, we can take a few minutes tonight to generate a list of things that you can do to boost your mood, pull yourself back up, or take care of yourself in some way. The thing is, when we are feeling overwhelmed, it is hard to think about fun things to do, because it just doesn't fit with our mood. It's much better to try to come up with a list for yourself ahead of time, and to get in the habit of doing those things.

In fact, as we'll talk about, you can write a letter to yourself. "Dear Self, if you are reading this, you are probably feeling overwhelmed. It is very important that you do one of the activities listed below. I know you don't feel like it right now, but trust me, you've got to just do it anyway." Or you can share your plan with a friend that you trust, who can say, "You know, you seem like you are getting down a little bit, let's go have some ice cream," or whatever it may be. Of course, it's not a good idea to eat ice cream all day long, but the idea is to do something actively to bring your mood back up.

I was talking to someone just today, struggling with depression, who has a pile of a month and a half of letters and bills sitting on her dining room table. She just throws it down, because she doesn't want to deal with it, and what's one more day? And then suddenly, it's a month and a half of stuff to go through, so why even bother? So her mood just keeps slipping down farther and farther. To break the cycle, you need to just pick some small thing and get moving, like, "I'm going to open up three pieces of mail today." You won't suddenly feel like, "Hooray, I love paying bills," but at least there will be a sense of, "Oh, good, I got something taken care of." That's a step up, where you are doing something that gives you that sense of mastery or satisfaction or accomplishment. You also need to do something pleasant for yourself, because again, part of the definition of depression is this low self-esteem that kicks in. Thoughts come up like, "I don't feel like taking a hot bath," or "I don't deserve to do something nice for myself." By paying attention, and catching it early, we can remind ourselves, "I don't feel like it right now, but I need to do this to take care of myself anyway."

Any questions or comments on that?

Kevin: I've already started on the list.

Dr. Sears: Good. Let's go ahead and take just a couple of minutes right now to write down a few things for yourself that are pleasurable, as well as some things that give you that accomplishment feeling. Again, you don't have to show this to anybody, and this is going to be part of your homework, but go ahead and jot some down for a few minutes just to get your list started.

Christine: For any day, any time?

Dr. Sears: It's great to have the longer-term goals, like going to Europe or something, but it is important to do little things on a daily basis. It can be lots of different things, and everybody here can have a completely different list. What one person might think is fun, another person might think is unbearable. Just try to come up with a few things you can do for yourself.

[pause]

Again, you can work on those more later as part of the homework. It's amazing how often people draw a blank when I ask them, "What do you do for fun, or hobbies, or to take care of yourself?" Especially if you are a parent, or very busy at work, you can have this mentality that, "I've got to get stuff done." It's an important shift to realize that you can still get things done and take care of yourself, like Laura was saying earlier.

So if we look at the handout, the theme for today is, "How can I best take care of myself?" In our culture, even to ask that question might be considered selfish, because we're told we should think more about others' needs. There is often a gender bias there, too, with women expected to be caretakers. You may have also internalized expectations when you were growing up, like always getting the work done first. So even just to give yourself permission to ask, "How can I take care of myself?" may be a big deal.

The next page is about using the breathing space—the action step. We talked about the three-minute breathing space, getting in touch with what is happening right now. And I think people have been asking, appropriately so, now what? I'm noticing here's what's going on, or I'm noticing pain, or I'm stressed out, or whatever. The fourth step of the three-minute breathing space is called the action step. "I'm tuned in. Now what am I going to do? Now that I know what is happening, where do I go from here?"

First of all, you could take some considered action. You may need to speak up about something, or there may be some physical action you need to do. You are more likely to make wise choices because you are more conscious and less reactive. You could also decide to do nothing, to just sit with it, and watch to see if it changes, or even passes on its own.

However, if strong emotions and thoughts are gripping me, and there is nothing I can directly do about the situation that is causing them, I can ask, "What do I need for myself right now? How can I best take care of myself?" So, here are three concrete categories of things you can do.

One thing you can do is something pleasurable, either by being kind to your body, or by engaging in enjoyable activities. The handout gives examples like take a nap, have a nice hot bath, treat yourself to your favorite food, a hot drink, facial, manicure, go for a walk, visit a friend, do a hobby. And again, this is very individualized. Gardening sounds like a lot of work to me, but other people love being outside, feeling the dirt, and watching things grow. It's definitely up to you to choose what gives you nourishment.

The second thing you can do is something that gives you a sense of mastery, satisfaction, achievement, or control. Accomplishing something. Clean the house, or if that's overwhelming, clean a part of the house, clean out a cupboard or a drawer. It's especially important to congratulate yourself when you complete a task, or part of a task, and to break it down into smaller steps.

	Otherwise, you can fall into, I'm trying to decide if I should say it out loud, I call it the "F★★★-it Effect." "What's the point? It's overwhelming! Why even bother?" I guess I could call it the "Chuck-it Effect." [laughter]
Laura:	The first one is more appropriate!
Dr. Sears:	So it's about getting moving, starting some momentum. When I had my own martial arts school, I was teaching five nights a week, and had a full-time job on top of that. Many days I would think, "I'm tired, I don't feel like it, I don't want to go. But I'm the instructor." And every single time, once I got there and started moving, it was fun. I was glad I went, I got exercise, people were enjoying it. So it can be important to remember, "I've just got to start. And then it's usually never as bad as I think it's going to be in my mind."
Kevin:	I need some advice with that, because one of the things that is on my daily list to do is clear out boxes from my whole lifetime that are just sitting in my parents' garage and cluttering things up. I've actually got it in my phone every day. One box, just do one box. I don't.
Laura:	You don't? It's too overwhelming to even do one?
Kevin:	I don't even do one box. And I know what you are saying is true. Once I start doing it, it isn't bad at all. What's the big deal? But I still don't do it. I still don't do it.
Dr. Sears:	We build it up in our minds. With mindfulness you can just check in with yourself when that happens. "Isn't this interesting—I know it would be good to empty a box, but I feel this resistance. Where am I feeling it? What is that about? Is there a thought in there?" You can kind of sit with that, and even choose not to open the box. You can first approach it from a place of noticing.
Kevin:	Okay.
Dr. Sears:	The third thing we can do as an action step to take care of ourselves is to act mindfully, or to come more into the moment. Chances are, if you are stressed, anxious, or depressed, you'll be feeling trapped in your thinking. So this is just saying, "Find something to pay attention to with your senses." Coming back to this moment. Walking down the stairs, you can feel the banister under your hand, you can feel the pressure of your shoes as you walk. Noticing what you are doing, as you are doing it. You could do that with noticing the food you are eating, or you could burn some incense, or smell some potpourri, really anything that brings you into your senses in the moment.
	On the next page, there are three points to remember about the things we're talking about. One is to do this as an experiment. Just like with all of the exercises, we are fostering an attitude of, "Let's just see what is happening. Let's just notice what happens." Try not to prejudge how you will feel after it's done. Just keep an

open mind, and know it may or may not be helpful, but keep an openness to experience.

The second thing is to consider a range of activities, not limiting yourself to a favorite few. Especially for depression, just trying something different, exploring and inquiring, works to counter the tendency to retreat and withdraw.

Number three is don't expect miracles. Just try it out as best you can. Don't put extra pressure on yourself, like, "I did this but I don't feel better. I'm such a loser, I can't even take a bath and feel better." Just recognize that no matter how you're feeling, no matter what your thoughts are, you can still choose what activity you want to do. Because otherwise, your whole life is driven by your feelings and by your thoughts, and you are not in charge of your life direction. This certainly may not be easy at times. I could feel horribly sad, but I can choose to take a walk instead of sit in the corner and fight it. Recognize that you may have a little more flexibility in your choices than you think at first.

Next in the handout are some suggestions for what to do if depression becomes overwhelming. Reminding yourself, "Just because I am depressed now doesn't mean I always will be." Recognizing the thoughts that are coming up, using the same skills you've already learned to get yourself through these worst periods.

Any thoughts, questions?

Kevin: I've noticed that there might be an activity on our list of things to do to feel good or to enjoy, but sometimes it depends on how you are feeling whether you are going to be able to get enjoyment out of it. Like this past Saturday, I did a half-day silent retreat, and it really was a good experience. And then, just out of the blue, I got hit with a really deep crying spell after the silent meditation. And I thought, man, I totally stayed with it, I didn't try to run away from it at all. Not at all. I totally let myself experience it, which was not pleasurable, but I totally let myself feel it. And then afterwards, I was like, "You know what, it still feels really, kind of heavy." I wanted to see if I can do something to feel a little better. I love cats, but I am not in a position where I can have a cat now, so I found out where an SPCA is, and I can go there, and just go in the rooms and play with the cats, pet the cats.

Laura: Cool! I didn't know you could do that.

Kevin: Totally! You just go in there and pet the cats, or dogs if you prefer. They also have rabbits. But that day, it didn't work at all. I went in there, pet cats a little bit, and I was like, "This isn't working." Rather than sit there and say, "Well, it's supposed to be working and it's not, so now I feel even worse, it's not working now, I'm going to leave."

Dr. Sears: I think that's a good attitude. That's also why we have a list of different things we can do. If you are prone to depression, you can slip into not doing anything, so the idea is to do *something*. So even if it doesn't make you feel better in that moment, it's better that you got out and did something actively, instead of just retreating and withdrawing. But yeah, that was a good attitude, "I thought I'd try it, it didn't seem to work like I wanted to, but . . ."

Kevin: Doesn't mean it won't work next time.

Dr. Sears: Yeah. And, "Oh, I'm noticing these thoughts coming up that 'it didn't work,' and 'I'm wasting my time.'" By noticing those, you are still making choices moment by moment.

So, we are only going to meet one more time. The last official home practice assignment. So number one is to think through all of the different exercises that we have done, and try to figure out what might be sustainable for you after the class is over. It is much better, even if it is relatively short, to have a regular, daily routine of some kind than to practice for several hours once a week or once month. Regularity in small doses seems to be better than big chunks intermittently. And it could be that every day you do something a little different. That's fine, just experiment for yourself and see what works for you.

The other two are to continue practicing the three-minute breathing space three times a day, and to practice remembering to do it in the middle of a stressful moment, or shortly after, to check in with yourself.

The last part is to come up with a relapse prevention plan. And again, this is just for you. You don't have to turn it in or show it to anybody else. We started talking about this earlier. First of all, recognizing, what are your personal warning signals that stress, anxiety, or depression are coming on very strong? A few examples are listed here in the handout, like becoming irritable, decreasing your social contact, changes in how you are sleeping or eating, feeling really exhausted, and giving up on exercise. Everyone will have their own unique set of warning signs.

The next part is to set up an early-warning system. Write down on a sheet of paper, again just for yourself, the changes you should watch out for. If you trust somebody close in your life, you can share it with them. People around us tend to notice more often or more quickly than we do. "I noticed you are getting a little irritable—how is your stress level?" The idea is to become more aware of when we're getting increasingly stressed, or depressed, or overwhelmed. Often, we want to pretend that it's not really happening, because we don't want to deal with it right then. Especially something like depression—it's so awful, you just don't want to believe it's really happening, so you just ignore it, or pretend it's not there, or withdraw to conserve your resources, which can make it worse. The important thing is to notice the warning signs that you are getting overwhelmed, and check in with yourself. You can then choose to do something to take care of yourself, and you are then in a better place to handle the situation.

So write down suggestions for an action plan that you can use for responding once you notice the warning signs. As I mentioned, you can write a letter to yourself. "Dear Richard—if you're reading this, it probably means you're getting overwhelmed. I know you don't feel like it right now, but it is very important that you do a couple of the activities listed below." It's hard to come up with a list of nourishing activities when you're feeling overwhelmed, so make your list while you're in a fairly good place.

At the very bottom of the page it says, "It may be helpful to remind yourself that what you need at times of difficulty is no different from what you have already practiced many times throughout this course" (Segal, Williams, & Teasdale, 2013, p. 361). We often fear we missed some important secret for dealing with challenges. All we are doing is practicing noticing, "Wow, I'm feeling really overwhelmed right now." We stay with it, and feel it, and then make a conscious choice, instead of falling into old, unhelpful reaction patterns.

All right, any other questions, thoughts? So, next time will be our last session!

12 Session 8

Extending New Learning

The last session provides an opportunity to reflect on the previous 7 weeks. Participants often note significant life changes. However, unless this momentum can be maintained through regular practice, it can be easy to fall back into old patterns. Creating and discussing plans and linking them to positive reasons for taking care of oneself is crucial for carrying the momentum forward.

The session begins with one of the first exercises done in the group, the body scan. The session ends with a brief meditation on a natural object and/or with wishing the other participants well. People enjoy keeping a small souvenir, like a stone, as a concrete reminder to notice the present moment. I also print a personal graduation certificate on fancy paper for each participant. This can provide documentation for mental health professionals but also acknowledges the commitment each person made to completing the group. I once had a very busy CEO tearfully exclaim that she was going to proudly hang it in her office.

Session 8 Transcript

Dr. Sears: So we made it to the last class!
Laura: I can't believe it's the last one already!
Dr. Sears: Are there any burning questions or comments? Well, we are kind of coming full circle in a way, so we are going to return to one of the ones we first did, our old friend the body scan.

[Body Scan Meditation]

Dr. Sears: Anybody want to guess how long that was?
Laura: Half an hour?
Dr. Sears: Yes, just about.
Christine: At one point I almost dozed off.
Dr. Sears: I was very aware of the stillness in the room. To me it's impressive that after only a few weeks you all have the ability to just sit still and be present with yourselves. Even if 90% of the time your mind is wandering, that's all right, you've learned to let that

	process happen and just be okay with it. Not that you have to sit still, but it's a sign that your mind is calm. It's just interesting to see the progress compared to the first day.
Laura:	The first time we did that, how long was it?
Dr. Sears:	I probably tried to keep it more like 20 minutes the first time. I'm already going off into the past—anybody want to comment on what they noticed during this exercise, or what their experience was?
Christine:	Well, very relaxed.
Stephanie:	When you said something about remembering the first time we were here, our first class, the similarities and the differences, I became aware of being very grateful that I have had this class at this time. It's really helped me through some tough stuff. A week ago, my husband, we are still living in the same house, put a fire in the fireplace. I had gone to let the dog out, and I was in the present moment, because I was aware of the cold air and the smell of the fireplace. Then it was like someone was burning something outside, and I came in and said, "It really smells like fall out there." But there was something that didn't quite set with that, and I kind of didn't judge it or whatever. Well, five minutes later, he comes through there and goes, "Call 911! There's something wrong!" And the fireplace—the smoke was just pouring out of the top of the house. I started to really panic, because my house burned to the ground when I was eight. So I realized I went into panic mode, but as I dialed 911, and it rang five times, I realized I was kind of taking a breath with every ring. I just said a small prayer, "God, help me," and all of a sudden this thought came, "Put the fire that's in the fireplace out!" It was just a thought, and I was like, "Oh my gosh! We have a fire extinguisher in our pantry!" I ran and grabbed it, and said, "Let's put the fire in the fireplace out!" The fire was contained within the chute, but it scorched the wall, it was in the top someplace. But if we hadn't done that, it probably would have been worse—they said, "Somehow, you managed to contain it." That was a gift. And it came from being present, and breathing. I was just waiting there, didn't have anything to do, and was kind of counting my breaths, and then I just said a quick prayer, a "God, help me." I just wanted to share that.
Dr. Sears:	Amazing!
Christine:	What are your thoughts on guided imagery? I tried it once or twice this past week, and I find it to be helpful, because it goes a step beyond just being aware. Is that something that you recommend?
Dr. Sears:	Sure. It's done in different ways. I'd be interested to know what you did.
Christine:	I have one that is for fatigue. It guides what your thoughts are, versus having no thoughts. Thinking about mindfulness of your body, or space around you.

Kevin:	Is it like "You are lying in a field. . ."?
Christine:	Sort of, and for me it's more helpful because I can think of the imagery that the person is guiding me with. There's more there than just your feelings of the present moment. It's guiding you to feel a certain way with fatigue or pain. I have a couple of them, and it takes it a step beyond. I mean I think it is helpful to obviously be mindful, and to maybe use that with the guided imagery. I think it is more helpful than the body scan by itself.
Dr. Sears:	By all means, experiment, and if it works, that's the test.
Christine:	It's more targeted towards different problems.
Dr. Sears:	I also see things like that as working together. If you were training in a traditional Asian monastery, you would start with mindfulness, to develop your attention, awareness, and concentration. And then, you could go on to all of these complicated practices, but it would be hard, for instance, to visualize something if your mind wanders too much.
Christine:	On the CD, when you talk about looking at your thoughts as leaves floating by, for me, that by itself calms my system down. That's why I thought maybe I should go back to the guided imagery, and see what happens. One of the ones I listen to has soft music in the background.
Laura:	How long is it? Is it like 15 or 30 minutes?
Christine:	Yeah, it's like 15 minutes. One's a little bit longer.
Dr. Sears:	This might sound like I'm selling mindfulness, but I also think you can get more out of those because you are doing them more consciously. "I'm going to choose to do this to deal with this pain." Otherwise, you can fall into, "Oh, I don't like the way I'm feeling, so I'm going to imagine I'm on a beach somewhere," which is a subtle way of avoiding what's uncomfortable. It sounds like you're using visualization as a way to engage with your experiences, and consciously choosing what tool to use. Adding more tools to the toolbox is important, too. I don't want you to come away thinking that you have to be mindful all the time. Use whatever works for you. The whole idea is just to bring more awareness, which gives you more conscious choice.
Christine:	It was interesting to go back to it, having had this class, to be more mindful.
Laura:	Did it seem to work better now?
Christine:	Yes! If you want to try it, I imagine you can look online for guided imagery, or ask someone here at the store to help you.
Dr. Sears:	Other experiences from the last week? One of the things was to think about early warning signs and action plans so you can help yourself when things start to get overwhelming, and coming up with a list of pleasant and mastery activities. And to experiment

with a mindfulness routine that is inspiring, or works well for you, that you can continue after the course.

Laura: I like the idea of, if you see warning signs, finding ways to not be pulled down. Because the past couple of years, I've always felt like I should be doing something. I need to be accomplishing something, and if I'm not doing work, then I'm being lazy. But yet, I still don't do it, I just feel bad. Like, "I'm going to bake some cupcakes," but I never do that. It might seem silly, but it's okay to give yourself permission to do self-care.

Dr. Sears: Yes, I like that phrase, "give yourself permission." This is the way I'm feeling, and just noticing it more. If I feel guilty, is this appropriate? Maybe it's just old stuff. When I was a kid, my mother would teasingly say, "If laziness hurt, you would scream all day!" [laughter]. We can be raised with a sense of, "There is so much to do, I don't have time for myself." Or if you're in school, there's always another assignment to do. Some jobs, you can feel like you're done at the end of the day, but a lot of jobs, it's like you are never finished. It's just constant.

Laura: I feel like I have a hard time separating work and the rest of my life. I'm always thinking about, "After this, I have to go back to my office and do some stuff." I'd rather just go home.

Dr. Sears: So now, you'll have a little more awareness, and you can decide, "I think I want to go to the office, because it will be good to get some work off my mind," or, "This feels like a compulsive thing, and it's never going to be done anyway, I can give myself permission to go home." It's totally up to you what you want to do. If you decide to go home, you can feel the guilt, and know that it will pass. Otherwise, you may only work to avoid guilt, or if you go home, it's like you're burning yourself up with the wasted energy of guilt, and don't enjoy being home anyway.

Laura: Yes, that's exactly how I feel!

Dr. Sears: Zen master Seung Sahn, before Nike came up with it, would say, "Just do it, or don't do it." Just decide. You hear this in lots of different ways. In *The Karate Kid*, Pat Morita said, "Right side of road, okay. Left side of road, okay. Middle, sooner or later, crushed like grape." Sometimes it is just better to make a decision, rather than being frozen with indecisiveness and getting neither choice. Of course, there's a balance. You don't necessarily want to jump into everything, either.

Laura: I'm very indecisive. I haven't figured out why. Sometimes I get frozen—it's silly things. I'm going out, and I can't figure out what to wear, and I'm late because of this inability to make a decision. "Pick something and put it on!" What causes us to get frozen in indecision?

Dr. Sears: There's probably a lot there, but now that you've got a little more awareness, you can just start with noticing. "What am I feeling as this is going on? Is there some worry about rejection? Maybe I just don't care?" There could be lots of things. It could be different every time.

We often say, "I want freedom, I want to do whatever I want, I want a choice." But making a choice can be paralyzing, because sometimes when I make a choice, it cuts off other possibilities. If I take this partner, then I can't have that partner. If I take this job, I can't be doing that job. We often want to keep all of our options open, so we're afraid to make a decision.

Or you decide, but then spend your time thinking, "What if I had chosen something else?" Now that you notice a little bit more, you can just decide and go from there.

Kevin: Sometimes, I find myself, I call it ruminating, sometimes I get a little message that says, "You know what? It doesn't matter." When the "doesn't matter" comes, that's easier. "Grab that!"

Christine: You don't always get that message. You need somebody to send it to us.

Kevin: You don't always get that message, no.

Dr. Sears: Yes, it's balance, too. Now I'm thinking about what my wife said this morning, "Are you going to wear those pants? They look a little wrinkled." Because normally, I don't care. There they are, they are easy and convenient. So, just noticing what's going on.

Kevin: But your shirt is perfect!

Dr. Sears: Thanks! But I think the more aware we become, the more freedom we have in choosing. "What I wear is really important, I am going to take some time to do this," or "Maybe the real thing is, I'm concerned what people will think about me when I get there."

Stephanie: Or, "I don't really want to go."

Dr. Sears: So instead of subconsciously delaying, you can just decide, "I'm not going to go, and I'll be okay with that." Or, "I know I'm going to feel guilty about not going for a little while, but I'm going to have a great time after the guilt goes away." So, more options. Anything else about the week, before we move on to the next thing?

So for the next part, pair up with the person next to you and take a few minutes to reflect back on the course. What your expectations were, what you learned, if you felt like there was something you didn't get, whatever seems relevant. And then we can talk about anything you want to share with the rest of the group.

[Partner Activity—reflecting on the course]

Dr. Sears: While it's fresh in your mind, if you're willing, the last page of the handout is a feedback form. There's a place to give a rating for how helpful the class has been, and anything you want to say about it.

[pause]

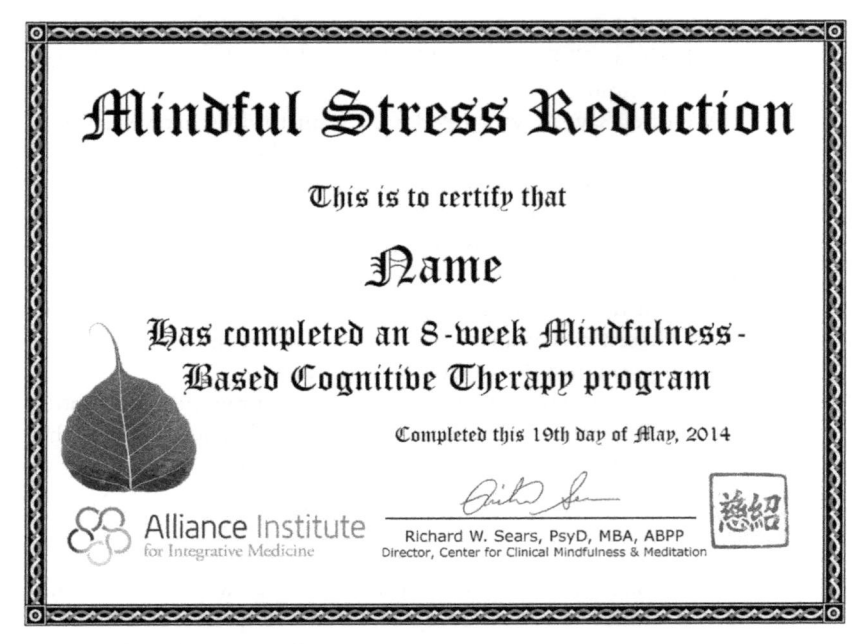

Figure 12.1 Graduation certificate

Dr. Sears: While you're doing that, here are your completion certificates!

[pause]

Dr. Sears: So, anybody have something they'd like to share with the larger group, anything that really stood out for you over the last eight weeks?

Stephanie: I thought it was very nice that whenever I came in and said I had done a terrible job with my homework, that you didn't put any pressure, you were like, "It's good that you noticed that." [laughter]

Laura: Celebrate the journey!

Stephanie: And that made it a lot easier for the next week to just do it.

Dr. Sears: Good, I'm glad to hear that. That is consciously what I was trying to do. To be transparent, I want to strongly encourage regular practice, because obviously the more you do it, the more you understand it, the more you get out of it. But just as you said, if it becomes this "thing you have to do," then it builds up resistance, or you quit, or you feel like it's not worth it.

Stephanie: Absolutely, or it was, I just felt awful. It was interesting, because I almost didn't go to that class that night, because I didn't want to. I failed!

Dr. Sears: To me, that's more what this is about, just noticing more and more things as they come up. "How interesting that it takes me a while to find clothes," or "How curious that I am not finishing this." I was talking to somebody today about that. "Here is my to-do list, I'll do that and that, but this one has been on my list for three weeks, and I should have done it a long time ago." Just to sit with that, and see what it brings up. "I wonder what that's about?" Just bringing more curiosity to it.

Stephanie: Last week, whenever I missed the class, I had been procrastinating on getting all of the financial stuff together to send to our attorneys. I'd been procrastinating and procrastinating, and I finally just sat down and said, "I am just going to do it." And I was just so focused on that. And it was like, "I am going to knock this out!" And I looked up, and it was 7:50 p.m., and I was like, "I missed my class!" And I was really shocked, so I guess it kind of helped me focus.

Dr. Sears: Yes, because there is a difference between, "I'm doing something important and I didn't get to it," versus a feeling of avoidance, like, "I don't want to do that because I know it's going to be unpleasant."

Laura: I think there's a book, or an essay, about procrastination that's called, "Eat the frog." If you eat a frog first thing, you get it over with, and you can go on with the rest of your day. Whatever you are procrastinating is the frog. Just eat the frog and get it over with.

Dr. Sears: I remember when that first dawned on me. It may sound funny since I like to give presentations now, but when I was in junior high school, I didn't want to present and stand in front of everybody. I would wait and go last. Then the time ran out, "Whew, missed it today!" Then I'd worry about it through the next class. I finally realized, if I go first, I can relax for the whole class. I don't know why it took me so long to figure that out. But again, it doesn't mean from now on, I've got to go first, and beat myself up and think I'm not good enough if I don't. It's just noticing, "This really does bother me, and I'm consciously avoiding it." We often try to fool ourselves with procrastination. "I'm going to go empty out this drawer because it's been bugging me," but you know you are only doing that to avoid something. It's okay to say, "I want to avoid that right now, so I'm going to go do this." It's compulsive, automatic procrastination that gets us into the most trouble.

Laura: I get tons of stuff done when I'm avoiding something else. [laughter]

Stephanie: I find I avoid stuff because sometimes I'm afraid I'm not going to do it perfectly. Sort of like picking out the perfect outfit.

Dr. Sears: So now, you have some more awareness, for good or for bad. "Why do I keep feeling like I want to do this perfectly? Maybe I'm just feeling some sadness, and if I focus on doing something perfectly, it distracts me from the feeling in there. Maybe if I sit with this feeling, I won't feel so driven to distract myself with unattainable perfection." It's fine to want to do things well, but the compulsive feelings actually detract from your ability to focus in the moment, and, ironically, impede you from doing things well.

Stephanie: That's interesting.

Dr. Sears: Anything else that you wanted to share?

Now let's discuss how you can keep your momentum going. The value of doing this as a group is you've got others to inspire you and share your experiences with. But since the group is ending, it's possible to slip back into old patterns of automatic pilot if you don't keep up regular practice.

Kevin: Yeah, I'm not a person of routine, I'm just not. I know myself. So it is very unlikely that I would set three specific times through the day to do the breathing or something like that. It's just not how I'm programmed. I hope you do organize a refresher course or periodic gathering. I would make it a priority. That would help me anchor it, for sure, and to continue it, and keep it fresh, and keep it in the forefront.

Dr. Sears: That's good to hear, because I have been getting reminders from the staff here. They are very supportive. It's just a matter of me committing the times to do it. That's one of those things I'm procrastinating [laughter].

There are places like churches, temples, or Zen centers where you can go for silent meditation practice, but not everyone is comfortable with the religious formalities that sometimes go along with that. There aren't a lot of secular places where you can just sit and be with yourself. You all know what I'm talking about. Your friends will ask, "What are you going to do for lunch?"

"I'm going to go sit with a bunch of people."

"Yeah, and do what?"

"I'm just going to sit and notice my thoughts, emotions, and body sensations."

"What? That's weird!"

Stephanie: "Have you been smoking pot?!" [laughter]

Dr. Sears: Another piece about keeping up momentum is that consistency is more important than quantity. As we talked about last week, it's better to do shorter exercises all through the week than to sit for hours only on the weekends. It's also important to set your intentions, clarifying that you will use this time for being present. If walking is my mindfulness practice, I'm going to feel the walking, and notice the trees around me, rather than spinning off in my head compulsively. And if I do spin off compulsively, I just notice that, and come back to the leaves on the trees that I see. Because, let's face it, this course has hopefully been a good experience, but it's only been eight weeks. It can be easy to fall back into older, deeply ingrained habits that you've practiced for years.

Kevin:	That's what you were saying, right? You were worried that you would go back to how things were.
Laura:	Right.
Dr. Sears:	I think there's a piece that makes the practice self-sustaining, meaning that, like you said, you noticed if you just take a few breaths, "Wow, I feel better!" And because you feel better, you are more likely to keep doing it. It's important not to make this drudgery. "I've had such a busy day, and now I've got to go sit." Maybe you won't be saying, "I can't wait to do my body scan tonight!", but hopefully, you can look forward to an exercise that represents your self-care time.

Books, audios, and videos about mindfulness theories and practices can also keep up motivation. As I've mentioned before, anything by Jon Kabat-Zinn is really good. There's a really thick book called *Coming to Our Senses* (Kabat-Zinn, 2006). Each chapter is only a couple of pages, so you can get in the habit of just reading one chapter each day, which will inspire you to sit.

We're short on time, so let's go through the handout, and then we'll have our last exercise. Looking at that initial page, the whole point of this is to take what we have been learning and apply it in your life. I hope you've been able to start doing that, as opposed to, "Now I have another thing I have to do." The whole point is to bring it into your life.

You have all probably heard the serenity prayer, which is a good model of what this course is about. The things I can change, give me the courage to change them, the things I can't change, let me accept them. And then the hard part, how do I know the difference between what I have to accept and what I can change? The space that we create with mindfulness can help with that.

The next page is about daily mindfulness, ways you can do mindfulness from moment to moment. Again, it doesn't have to be a separate thing from your life. Here are some more ways of bringing it in.

On the last page, I list a few websites and book titles. I also list some sources for more audio of mindfulness exercises. Jon Kabat-Zinn of course has some wonderful CDs.

Laura:	Is that his voice on track 5 of your CD, on loving-kindness?
Dr. Sears:	That's my friend, Dennis Tirch (Sears, Tirch, & Denton, 2011).
Laura:	I love that one. I listened to that for the first time this week, and his voice is just so soothing.
Dr. Sears:	Oh, good. I enjoy his recording also. Okay, any other comments or questions? What I'd like you to do for our last exercise is take one stone out of this bag . . .
Laura:	I thought it was candy.

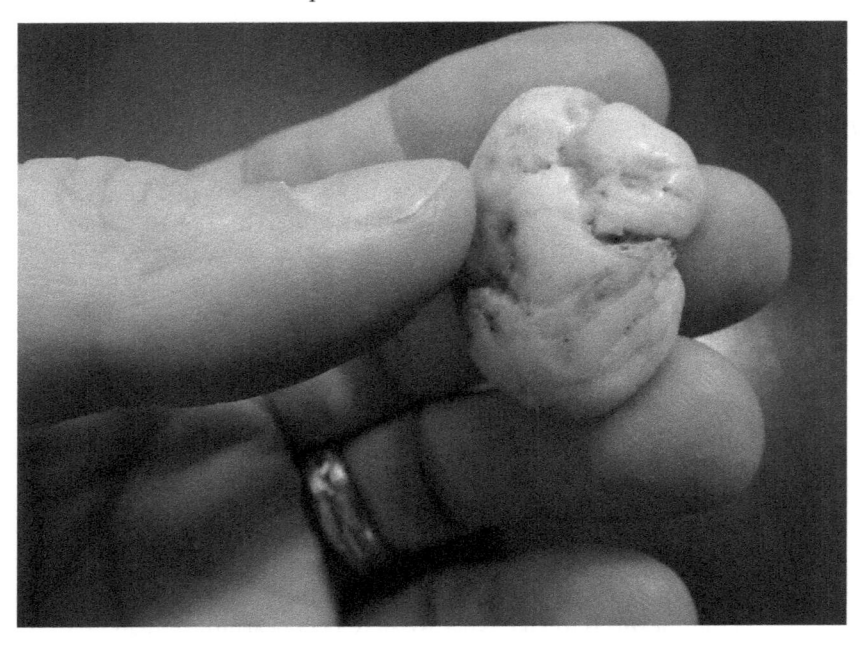

Figure 12.2 Rock exercise

Kevin: Yogurt-covered raisins.
Dr. Sears: You're not going to have to put this in your mouth! [laughter]

[Rock exercise]

So whenever you are ready, bringing your attention back to the rest of the room.

You are welcome to keep this stone. Some people have told me they like to keep it in their pocket, or put it on their desk or something, as just a little reminder to pay more attention. It's something solid and concrete you can squeeze in your hand when you find yourself getting lost in thoughts. Kind of a reminder of this class and a connection to what we've been practicing together. Any comments on this exercise?

Stephanie: I was aware, when we picked them up, they were cold.
Dr. Sears: They were in my car.
Stephanie: It's really warm now. It's interesting.
Dr. Sears: Anything else on that exercise, or any final wise comments or questions? Again, I do plan to do the ongoing groups, but otherwise, you all have my e-mail on the handouts if you have questions along the way or just want to stay in touch.

I also want to say that I'm honored that all of you came here. You committed a lot of your life to being here, and shared a lot with me. I really do grow from all of the experiences and energy

|||||||||||||||||||||||||||||||||||||||||||||||||||||||||||||||||||||||||||||||||||

	that you bring into this, so it's an honor to be able to share this with you. It takes a lot of trust, too, to come in here and do this. Like in the video, "It was weird when you made us eat a raisin the first session." So it means a lot to me that you all came. I really appreciate all of you being here, and I hope you will stay in touch.
Kevin:	Thanks, man, it was great.
Stephanie:	I've enjoyed everyone, too. It's been a good group. Thank you.
Dr. Sears:	People sometimes ask me if they can do this privately, but it never seems to work as well. There is just something about doing it with other people that makes it more useful—hopefully all of you had that experience.
Stephanie:	Oh, absolutely!
Dr. Sears:	Being able to share and listen to all the different perspectives, and discuss how it's working for you. It helps to get some validation, and to realize you're not alone on your journey.
Stephanie:	And Laura, you shared some things that were really powerful. When you shared about your parents, that was just amazing to me. Thank you.
Laura:	You're welcome.

Participant Feedback Forms

After reflecting on the entire course, participants are asked to provide written feedback while it is fresh in their minds. The responses of the members of this group are provided below.

On a scale of 1–10, how important has this program been for you?
10, 8, 8, 8
Please say why you have given it this rating.

Participant 1

I feel this program was very important for me at this point in my life. I believe it has helped me through the past 2 months in so many ways.

That being said, I also realize that I need to address discipline and procrastination issues. I got so much out of the homework *when* I actually did it.

You were great and I appreciate the way you made it easy to get honest and be open with my truth and what I was experiencing.

Participant 2

This course has given me a foundation for finding ways to deal with my anxiety. I didn't know how to get started with meditation and this definitely helped! I probably would have gotten more out of it if I had done all of the homework, but I still learned a lot and was able to incorporate it into my daily life.

Thanks!

Participant 3

We're dealing here with nothing less than the content of one's own thoughts! It's a long journey to step back and observe one's thoughts—that they're not "real" but just ephemeral. The 8-week course may be the tip of the iceberg in my process of "weeding out" thoughts and patterns which are unhelpful.

I do hope we have a periodic gathering, as that will help a lot to keep the work present for me. I'm not a person of routine, so anchoring the work into a daily schedule is unlikely for me.

I do think the timing of the course was good for me, and I enjoyed it a lot. The homework sheets will serve as a memoir of this 2-month difficult period that I've been dealing with high anxiety.

Participant 4

It's been helpful to become more mindful of thoughts and feelings, as well as my body's physical response to situations (both positive and negative). I found the class became more effective for me personally, when we started to discuss what to do with that heightened sensitivity/awareness to pain, stress, fatigue, etc.

I enjoyed the open discussion and felt that I could share whatever thoughts I had.

Thanks!

References

Albers, S. (2003). *Eating mindfully: How to end mindless eating and enjoy a balanced relationship with food*. Oakland, CA: New Harbinger Publications, Inc.

Allen, M., Bromley, A., Kuyken, W., & Sonnenberg, S. (2009). Participants' experiences of mindfulness-based cognitive therapy: "It changed me in just about every way possible." *Behavioural Cognitive Psychotherapy, 34*(4), 413–430.

American Psychiatric Association. (2000). *Diagnostic and statistical manual of mental disorders* (4th ed., text rev.). Washington, DC: Author.

American Psychological Association. (2002). Ethical principles of psychologists and code of conduct. *American Psychologist, 57*, 1060–1073.

American Psychological Association. (2003). Guidelines on multicultural education, training, research, practice, and organizational change for psychologists. *American Psychologist, 58*, 377–402.

American Psychological Association. (2007). Record keeping guidelines. *American Psychologist, 62*, 993–1004.

American Psychological Association. (2010). Guidelines for child custody evaluations in family law proceedings. *American Psychologist, 65*(9), 863–867. DOI: 10.1037/a0021250

Barnett, J. (2007). Positive ethics, risk management, and defensive practice. *The Maryland Psychologist, 53*(1), 30–31.

Bartley, T. (2011). *Mindfulness-based cognitive therapy for cancer*. London, UK: Wiley-Blackwell.

Beck, A. (1967). *Depression: Clinical, experimental, and theoretical aspects*. New York: Hoeber.

Bernard, J., & Goodyear, R. (2014). *Fundamentals of clinical supervision* (5th ed.). Upper Saddle River, NJ: Merrill.

Bögels, S., & Restifo, K. (2014). *Mindful parenting: A guide for mental health practitioners*. New York: Springer.

Bowen, S., Chawla, N., & Marlatt, A. (2010). *Mindfulness-based relapse prevention for addictive behaviors: A clinician's guide*. New York: Guilford Press.

Coelho, H., Canter, P., & Ernst, E. (2007). Mindfulness-based cognitive therapy: Evaluating current evidence and informing future research. *Journal of Consulting and Clinical Psychology, 75*(6), 1000–1005.

Collard, P. (2013). *Mindfulness-based cognitive therapy for dummies*. Chichester, West Sussex, UK: John Wiley & Sons.

Corey, G. (2012). *Theory and practice of group counseling* (8th ed.). Belmont, CA: Brooks/Cole, Cengage Learning.

Cotton, S., Luberto, C. M., Stahl, L., Sears, R. W., & DelBello, M. (2014, May). Mindfulness-based cognitive therapy for youth with anxiety disorders at risk for bipolar disorder: A pilot trial.

Presentation for the International Research Congress on Integrative Medicine and Health, Miami, FL.
Covey, S. (1989). *The seven habits of highly effective people: Restoring the character ethic.* New York: Simon and Schuster.
Crane, R. (2009). *Mindfulness-based cognitive therapy.* London and New York: Routledge.
Crane, R., Kuyken, W., Williams, M., Hastings, R., Cooper, L., & Fennell, M. (2012). Competence in teaching mindfulness-based courses: Concepts, development, and assessment. *Mindfulness, 3,* 76–84. DOI: 0.1007/s12671-011-0073-2
Davidson, R., Kabat-Zinn, J., Schumacher, J., Rosenkranz, M., Muller, D., Santorelli, S., Urbanowski, F., Harrington, A., Bonus, K., & Sheridan, J. (2003). Alterations in brain and immune function produced by mindfulness meditation. *Psychosomatic Medicine, 65*(4), 564–570.
Davis, D., & Hayes, H. (2011). What are the benefits of mindfulness? A practice review of psychotherapy-related research. *Psychotherapy, 48*(2), 198–208. DOI: 10.1037/a0022062
Davis, L., & Luedtke, B. (2013, August). *Introduction to mindfulness-based cognitive-behavioral conjoint therapy for PTSD.* Workshop presented at the APA Annual Convention, Honolulu, HI.
Deckersbach, T., Hölzel, B., Eisner, L., Lazar, S., & Nierenberg, A. (2014). *Mindfulness-based cognitive therapy for bipolar disorder.* New York: Guilford Press.
Dharma, W. (2010). *Five Mountain record: The kongan collection of the Five Mountain Order.* Kansas City, MO: Before Thought Publications.
Didonna, F. (Ed.). (2009). *Clinical handbook of mindfulness.* New York: Springer.
Duncan, L., & Bardacke, N. (2010). Mindfulness-based childbirth and parenting education: Promoting family mindfulness during the perinatal period. *Journal of Child & Family Studies, 19,* 190–202. DOI: 10.1007/s10826-009-9313-7
Falender, C., & Shafranske, E. (2004). *Clinical supervision: A competency-based approach.* Washington, DC: American Psychological Association.
Farb, N., Segal, Z., & Anderson, A. (2013). Mindfulness meditation training alters cortical representations of interoceptive attention. *Social, Cognitive & Affective Neuroscience, 8,* 15–26.
Farb, N., Segal, Z., Mayberg, H., Bean, J., McKeon, D., & Anderson, A. (2007). Mindfulness training reveals dissociable neural modes of self-reference. *Social, Cognitive and Affective Neuroscience, 2,* 313–322.
Finucane, A., & Mercer, S. (2006). An exploratory mixed-methods study of the acceptability and effectiveness of mindfulness-based cognitive therapy for patients with active depression and anxiety in primary care. *BMC Psychiatry, 6,* 1–14.
Foa, E., Hembree, E., & Rothbaum, B. (2007). *Prolonged exposure therapy for PTSD: Emotional processing of traumatic experiences: Therapist guide.* Oxford: Oxford University Press.
Fouad, N., Gerstein, L., & Toporek, R. (2006). Social justice and counseling psychology in context. In R. Toporek, L. Gerstein, N. Fouad, G. Roysircar, & T. Israel (Eds.), *Handbook for Social Justice in Counseling Psychology* (pp. 1–16). Thousand Oaks, CA: Sage Publications.
Fuchs, C., Lee, J., Roemer, L., & Orsillo, S. (2013). Using mindfulness-and acceptance-based treatments with clients from nondominant cultural and/or marginalized backgrounds: Clinical considerations, meta-analysis findings, and introduction to the special series: Clinical considerations in using acceptance- and mindfulness-based treatments with diverse populations. *Cognitive and Behavioral Practice, 20*(1), 1–12. DOI: http://dx.doi.org/10.1016/j.cbpra.2011.12.004
Fulton, P. (2005). Mindfulness as clinical training. In C. Germer, R. Siegel, & P. Fulton (Eds.), *Mindfulness and psychotherapy.* New York: Guilford Press.

Goleman, D., & Kabat-Zinn, J. (2007). *Mindfulness @ work* [Audio CD]. New York: MacMillan Audio.

Greenberger, D., & Padesky, C. (1995). *Mind over mood: A cognitive therapy treatment manual for clients*. New York: Guilford Press.

Grepmair, L., Mietterlehner, F., Loew, T., Bachler, E., Rother, W., & Nickel, N. (2007). Promoting mindfulness in psychotherapists in training influences the treatment results of their patients: A randomized, double-blind, controlled study. *Psychotherapy and Psychosomatics, 76*, 332–338. DOI: 10.1159/000107560

Gunaratana, H. (2011). *Mindfulness in plain English*. Boston: Wisdom Publications.

Guthrie, R. (2003). *Even the rat was white: A historical view of psychology* (2nd ed.). Boston: Allyn & Bacon.

Harris, R. (2008). *The happiness trap: How to stop struggling and start living*. Boston: Trumpeter.

Hayes, S. (2007). Commentary: Language, self, and diversity. In J. Muran (Ed.), *Dialogues on difference: Studies of diversity in the therapeutic relationship* (pp. 275–279). Washington, DC: American Psychological Association. DOI: 10.1037/11500-030

Helms, J. (1992). *A race is a nice thing to have: A guide to being a white person or understanding the white persons in your life*. Topeka, KS: Content Communications.

Hofmann, S., Sawyer, A., Witt, A., & Oh, D. (2010). The effect of mindfulness-based therapy on anxiety and depression: A meta-analytic review. *Journal of Consulting and Clinical Psychology, 78*(2), 169–183.

Hollon, S., & Beck, A. (1986). Cognitive and cognitive-behavioral therapies. In A. Bergin & S. Garfield (Eds.), *Handbook of psychotherapy and behavior change* (3rd ed., pp. 446–448). New York: Wiley.

Hölzel, B., Lazar, S., Gard, T., Schuman-Olivier, Z., Vago, D., & Ott, U. (2011). How does mindfulness meditation work? Proposing mechanisms of action from a conceptual and neural perspective. *Perspectives on Psychological Science, 6*(6), 537–559. DOI: 10.1177/1745691611419671

Ingram, R., Atchley, R., & Segal, Z. (2011). *Vulnerability to depression: From cognitive neuroscience to prevention and treatment*. New York: Guilford Press.

Kabat-Zinn, J. (1994). *Wherever you go there you are*. New York: Hyperion.

Kabat-Zinn, J. (2003). Mindfulness-based interventions in context: Past, present, and future. *Clinical Psychology: Science and Practice, 10*(2), 144–156.

Kabat-Zinn, J. (2006). *Coming to our senses: Healing ourselves and the world through mindfulness*. New York: Hyperion.

Kabat-Zinn, J. (2010). *Mindfulness meditation for pain relief: Guided practices for reclaiming your body and your life* [audio CD]. Boulder, CO: Sounds True.

Kabat-Zinn, J. (2012). *Guided mindfulness meditation: Series 3* [audio CD]. Boulder, CO: Sounds True.

Kabat-Zinn, J. (2013). *Full catastrophe living: Using the wisdom of your body and mind to face stress, pain, and illness* (rev. ed.). New York: Bantam.

Kabat-Zinn, J., & Moyers, B. (1993). *Healing from within* [video]. New York: Ambrose Video. Episode of the Bill Moyers series, *Healing and the Mind*, that follows Jon Kabat-Zinn taking a group through the 8 weeks of an MBSR course.

Keller, M., Lavori, P., Lewis, C., & Klerman, G. (1983). Predictors of relapse in major depressive disorder. *JAMA, 250*, 3299–3304.

Krishnamurti, J. (2012). *Choiceless awareness*. Ojai, CA: Krishnamurti Foundation.

Kristeller, J., Baer, R., & Quillian, R. (2006). Mindfulness-based approaches to eating disorders. In R. A. Baer (Ed.), *Mindfulness and acceptance-based interventions: Conceptualization, application, and empirical support* (pp. 75–91). San Diego, CA: Elsevier.

Kristeller, J., & Wolever, R. (2011). Mindfulness-based eating awareness training for treating binge eating disorder: The conceptual foundation. *Eating Disorders, 19*(1), 49–61. DOI: 10.1080/10640266.2011.533605

Kupfer, D. (1991). Long-term treatment of depression. *Journal of Clinical Psychiatry, 52* Suppl. 28–34.

Kuyken, W., Byford, S., Byng, R., Dalgleish, T., Lewis, G., Taylor, R., Watkins, E., Hayes, R., Lanham, P., Kessler, D., Morant, N., & Evans, A. (2010). Study protocol for a randomized controlled trial comparing mindfulness-based cognitive therapy with maintenance antidepressant treatment in the prevention of depressive relapse/recurrence: the PREVENT trial. *BMC Trials, 11*, 99. DOI:10.1186/1745-6215-11-99

Kuyken, W., Crane, R., & Dalgleish, T. (2012). Does mindfulness-based cognitive therapy prevent depressive relapse? *British Medical Journal*, 345, e7194. DOI: 10.1136/bmj.e7194. Published online November 9, 2012.

Kuyken, W., Watkins, E., Holden, E., White, K., Taylor, R. S., Byford, S., ... Dalgleish, T. (2010). How does mindfulness-based cognitive therapy work? *Behaviour Research and Therapy, 48*(11), 1105–1112. DOI: 10.1016/j.brat.2010.08.003

Lazar, S., Kerr, C., Wasserman, R., Gray, J., Greve, D., Treadway, M., ... Fischl, B. (2005). Meditation experience is associated with increased cortical thickness. *Neuroreport, 16*(17), 1893–1897.

Leahy, R. (2003). *Cognitive therapy techniques: A practitioner's guide.* New York: Guilford Press.

Linehan, M. (1993). *Cognitive behavioral treatment of borderline personality disorder.* New York: Guilford Press.

Longmore, R., & Worrell, M. (2007). Do we need to challenge thoughts in cognitive behavior therapy? *Clinical Psychology Review, 27*, 173–187.

Ma, S., & Teasdale, J. (2004). Mindfulness-based cognitive therapy for depression: Replication and exploration of differential relapse prevention effects. *Journal of Consulting and Clinical Psychology, 72*, 31–40.

Mason, O., & Hargreaves, I. (2001). A qualitative study of mindfulness-based cognitive therapy for depression. *British Journal of Medical Psychology, 74*(2), 197–212.

Masuda, A. (2014). *Mindfulness and acceptance in multicultural competency: A contextual approach to sociocultural diversity in theory and practice.* Oakland, CA: New Harbinger Publications.

McBee, L. (2008). *Mindfulness-based elder care: A CAM model for frail elders and their caregivers.* New York: Springer.

McConnell, A., & Sears, R. (2014). Mindfulness in organizations. *Ohio Psychologist, 61,* 7–9.

McCown, D., Reibel, D., & Micozzi, M. (2011). *Teaching mindfulness: A practical guide for clinicians and educators.* New York: Springer.

McGrath, P. (2013, November). *Taking anxiety disorder treatment to the next level: Using exposure and response prevention for maximum effect.* 47th ABCT Annual Convention, Nashville, TN.

McMullin, R. (2000). *The new handbook of cognitive therapy techniques* (rev. ed.). New York: W.W. Norton.

Miller, W., & Rollnick, S. (2013). *Motivational interviewing: Helping people change* (3rd ed.). New York: Guilford Press.

Newberg, A., D'Aquili, E., & Rause, V. (2001). *Why God won't go away: Brain science and the biology of belief.* New York: Random House, Inc.

New Economics Foundation. (2008). Five ways to wellbeing. Downloaded July 8, 2014, from www.neweconomics.org/page/-/files/Five_Ways_to_Well-being_Evidence.pdf

Niemiec, R. (2014). *Mindfulness and character strengths: A practical guide to flourishing.* Boston: Hogrefe Publishing.

Piet, J., & Hougaard, E. (2011). The effect of mindfulness-based cognitive therapy for prevention of relapse in recurrent major depressive disorder: A systematic review and meta-analysis. *Clinical Psychology Review, 31*, 1032–1040.

Ponterotto, J., Casas, J., Suzuki, L., & Alexander, C. (2010). *Handbook of multicultural counseling* (3rd ed.). Los Angeles, CA: SAGE Publications.

Pope, K., & Tabachnick, B. (1993). Therapists' anger, hate, fear, and sexual feelings: National survey of therapist responses, client characteristics, critical events, formal complaints, and training. *Professional Psychology: Research and Practice, 24*, 142–152.

Pope, K., Tabachnick, B., & Keith-Spiegel, P. (1987). Ethics of practice: The beliefs and behaviors of psychologists as therapists. *American Psychologist, 42*, 993–1006.

Posner, M., & Rafal, R. (1986). Cognitive theories of attention and the rehabilitation of attentional deficits. In M. J. Meier, A. L. Benton, & L. Miller (Eds.), *Neuropsychological rehabilitation* (pp. 182–201). New York: Guilford Press.

Resick, P., Monson, C., & Chard, K. (2008). *Cognitive processing therapy veteran/military version: Therapist's manual*. Washington, DC: Department of Veteran's Affairs.

Sadlier, M., Stephens, S., & Kennedy, V. (2008). Tinnitus rehabilitation: A mindfulness meditation cognitive behavioural therapy approach. *Journal of Laryngology and Otology, 122*(1), 31–37.

Santorelli, S. (2000). *Heal thy self: Lessons on mindfulness in medicine*. New York: Crown Publishers.

Sapolsky, R. (2010). *Stress and your body* [audio CD]. Chantilly, VA: The Teaching Company.

Sears, R. (2012). *Mindfulness-based cognitive therapy: An introduction and overview* [video file]. Washington, DC: American Psychological Association.

Sears, R. (2014). *Mindfulness: Living through challenges and enriching your life in this moment*. London, UK: Wiley-Blackwell.

Sears, R., & Chard, K. (2015). *Mindfulness-based cognitive therapy for posttraumatic stress disorder*. London, UK: Wiley-Blackwell.

Sears, R., & Niblick, A. (Eds.). (2014). *Perspectives on religion and spirituality in psychotherapy*. Sarasota, FL: Professional Resource Press.

Sears, R., Rudisill, J., & Mason-Sears, C. (2006). *Consultation skills for mental health professionals*. New York: John Wiley & Sons.

Sears, R., Tirch, D., & Denton, R. (2011). *Mindfulness in clinical practice*. Sarasota, FL: Professional Resource Press.

Segal, Z. (2008). *Mindfulness-based cognitive therapy for depression and anxiety* [CD]. Lancaster, PA: J&K Seminars, LLC.

Segal, Z. (2013, November). *A day of mindful practice to enhance your clinical practice*. 47th ABCT Annual Convention, Nashville, TN.

Segal, Z., Bieling, P., Young, T. MacQueen, G., Cooke, R., Martin, L., Bloch, R., & Levitan, R. (2010). Antidepressant monotherapy versus sequential pharmacotherapy and mindfulness-based cognitive therapy, or placebo, for relapse prophylaxis in recurrent depression. *Archives of General Psychiatry, 67*, 1256–1264.

Segal, Z., & Carlson, J. (2005). *Mindfulness-based cognitive therapy for depression* [DVD]. Washington, DC: American Psychological Association.

Segal, Z., Gemar, M., & Williams, S. (1999). Differential cognitive response to a mood challenge following successful cognitive therapy or pharmacotherapy for unipolar depression. *Journal of Abnormal Psychology, 108*, 3–10.

Segal, Z., & Lau, M. (2013, November). *Mindfulness-based cognitive therapy for depression (2nd ed.): A clinical and research update*. 47th ABCT Annual Convention, Nashville, TN.

Segal, Z., Teasdale, & Williams, J. (2004). Mindfulness-based cognitive therapy: Theoretical rationale and empirical status. In S. Hayes, V. Follete, & M. Linehan (Eds.), *Mindfulness and acceptance* (pp. 45–65). New York: Guilford Press.

Segal, Z., Teasdale, J., Williams, M., & Gemar, M. (2002). The mindfulness-based cognitive therapy adherence scale: Inter-rater reliability, adherence to protocol and treatment distinctiveness. *Clinical Psychology & Psychotherapy, 9*(2), 131–138. DOI: 10.1002/cpp.320

Segal, Z., Williams, M., & Teasdale, J. (2002). *Mindfulness-based cognitive therapy for depression.* New York: Guilford Press.

Segal, Z., Williams, M., & Teasdale, J. (2013). *Mindfulness-based cognitive therapy for depression* (2nd ed.). New York: Guilford Press.

Selye, H. (1976). *Stress in health and disease.* Reading, MA: Butterworth's.

Semple, R., & Lee, J. (2011). *Mindfulness-based cognitive therapy for anxious children.* Oakland, CA: New Harbinger Publications, Inc.

Senge, P., Scharmer, C., Jaworski, J., & Flowers, B. (2004). *Presence: Human purpose and the field of the future.* Cambridge, MA: Society for Organizational Learning.

Shapiro, S., Brown, K., & Biegel, G. (2007). Teaching self-care to caregivers: Effects of mindfulness-based stress reduction on the mental health of therapists in training. *Training and Education in Professional Psychology, 1,* 105–115.

Siegel, D. (2007). *The mindful brain: Reflection and attunement in the cultivation of well-being.* New York: W. W. Norton & Company.

Smith, A., Graham, L., & Senthinathan, S. (2007). Mindfulness-based cognitive therapy for recurring depression in older people: A qualitative study. *Aging & Mental Health, 11*(3), 346–357.

Sohlberg, M., & Mateer, C. (1989). *Introduction to cognitive rehabilitation: Theory and practice.* New York: Guilford Press.

Sue, D., Capodilupo, C., Torino, G., Bucceri, J., Holder, A., Nadal, K., & Esquilin, M. (2007). Racial microaggressions in everyday life: Implications for clinical practice. *American Psychologist, 62*(4), 271–286. DOI: 10.1037/0003-066X.62.4.271

Surawy, C., McManus, M., Muse, K., & Williams, M. (2014). Mindfulness-based cognitive therapy (MBCT) for health anxiety (hypochondriasis): Rationale, implementation and case illustration. *Mindfulness, 21,* 1–11. DOI: 10.1007/s12671-013-0271-1

Teasdale J., Segal Z., & Williams, J. M. G. (1995). How does cognitive therapy prevent depressive relapse and why should attentional control (mindfulness) training help? *Behavioral Research and Therapy, 33,* 25–39.

Teasdale, J., Segal, Z., Williams, J. M. G., Ridgeway, V., Soulsby, J., & Lau, M. (2000). Prevention of relapse/recurrence in major depression by mindfulness-based cognitive therapy. *Journal of Consulting and Clinical Psychology, 68,* 615–623.

Teasdale, J., Williams, M., & Segal, Z. (2014). *The mindful way workbook: An 8-week program to free yourself from depression and emotional distress.* New York: Guilford Press.

Ting-Toomey, S. (2009). A mindful approach to managing conflict in intercultural intimate couples. In T. Karis & K. Killian (Eds.), *Intercultural couples: Exploring diversity in intimate relationships* (pp. 31–49). New York: Routledge/Taylor & Francis Group.

Ucros, G. (1989). Mood state-dependent memory: A meta-analysis. *Cognition & Emotion, 3*(2), 139–169. DOI: 10.1080/02699938908408077

UK Network for Mindfulness-Based Teacher Training Organisations. (2011). *Good practice guidelines for teaching mindfulness-based courses.* http://mindfulnessteachersuk.org.uk/pdf/teacher-guidelines.pdf

Vacarr, B. (2001). Moving beyond polite correctness: Practicing mindfulness in the diverse classroom. *Harvard Educational Review, 71*(2), 285–295.

Wegner, D., Schneider, D., Carter, S., & White, T. (1987). Paradoxical effects of thought suppression. *Journal of Personality and Social Psychology, 53,* 5–13.

Williams, J. M. G., & Kuyken, W. (2012). Mindfulness-based cognitive therapy: A promising new approach to preventing depressive relapse. *British Journal of Psychiatry, 200,* 359–360. DOI: 10.1192/bjp.bp.111.104745

Williams, K. (2006). Mindfulness-based stress reduction in a worksite wellness program. In R. Baer (Ed.), *Mindfulness-based treatment approaches: Clinician's guide to evidence base and applications* (pp. 361–375). Burlington, MA: Academic Press.

Williams, M. (2009). *Mindfulness-based cognitive therapy and the prevention of depression: Training video.* New York: Association for Behavioral and Cognitive Therapies. DVD video of Mark Williams covering basic principles of MBCT.

Williams, M., & Penman, D. (2011). *Mindfulness: An eight-week plan for finding peace in a frantic world.* Emmaus, PA: Rodale Books.

Williams, M., Teasdale, J., Segal, Z., & Kabat-Zinn, J. (2007). *The mindful way through depression: Freeing yourself from chronic unhappiness.* New York: Guilford Press.

Williams, M. J., McManus, M., Muse, K., & Williams, J. M. G. (2011). Mindfulness-based cognitive therapy for severe health anxiety (hypochondriasis): An interpretative phenomenological analysis of patients' experiences. *British Journal of Clinical Psychology, 50,* 379–397.

Woidneck, M., Pratt, K., Gundy, J., Nelson, C., & Twohig, M. (2012). Exploring cultural competence in acceptance and commitment therapy outcome research. *Professional Psychology: Research and Practice, 43,* 227–233.

Woods, S. (2010). *Mindfulness meditation with Susan Woods* [audio CDs]. Stowe, VT: Author.

Woods, S. (2013). Building a framework for mindful inquiry. www.slwoods.com

Woods, S. (2014). Training guidelines for MBCT teachers. www.slwoods.com

Yalom, I. (2006). *Understanding group psychotherapy: Volume 2, Inpatients* [DVD]. San Francisco, CA: Psychotherapy.net.

Yalom, I., & Leszcz, M. (2005). *The theory and practice of group psychotherapy* (5th ed.). New York: Basic Books.

Index

Note: page numbers in *italics* indicate figures.

ABC model 3–4, 89
absorption meditation 52, 57
acceptance 139, 141
acceptance and commitment therapy 1, 13
activating events 89
activity, well-being and 50
acupuncture 146
acutely depressed, MBCT and 36–7
addictions, MBCT and 4, 37–8, 56
advice givers/cotherapists, MBCT and 33–4
affect tolerance 1
allowing: overview 131–2; session transcript 132–44
antecedents 89
anxiety, MBCT and 37, 45–6, 56
applied learning: overview 175; session transcript 175–86
attention, kinds of 53–4
attitude 26–7
automatic pilot 71
automatic reactions 59
automatic thoughts 154
automatic thoughts questionnaire 125
aversion, recognizing: overview 116; session transcript 116–30
avoidance, relaxation methods and 58
avoidance cycles 27
awareness 53
awareness and autopilot: overview 63–4; session transcript 64–78
awareness training 24

barriers to mindfulness: overview 79; session transcript 79–96
beginner's mind 21
belief/behavior 89
bipolar disorder, MBCT and 4
body scan exercise 73–8, 79–83, 175

brain function 52
breath, mindfulness of: overview 97–8; session transcript 98–115
Buddha, the 52
business professionals, MBCT and 33
Byerly-Lamm, Karen 4

cancer, MBCT and 4
challenges: overview 79; session transcript 79–96
challenging participants: acutely depressed clients 36–7; addictions 37–8; advice givers/cotherapists 33–4; anxious clients 37; business professionals 33; eccentric clients 34–5; experienced mediators 34; groupies 36; health professionals 32; naysayers 35; overview 30–2; silent clients 36; stuck in the future 37; stuck in the past 36–7; traumas 38
challenging questions 64
Chard, Kate 23–4
children, MBCT for 14
choicefulness 1
choiceless awareness 20
chronic stress 49
clinical depression relapse statistics 2
cognitive-behavioral therapy (CBT) 2–4
cold water analogy 112
Coming to Our Senses (Kabat-Zinn) 183
completion certificates *180*
computer-projected presentation slides 46
confidentiality 64
connection, well-being and 50
consequences 89
constant learning, well-being and 51–2
content-related expertise 14
Covey, Stephen 89
crisis intervention mode 27

decentering process 3, 57
decoupling 28
"defusion" 57
depression, MBCT and 45–6, 57, 125–7, 168–9
depressive disorder 2
dialectical behavior therapy 1, 2
didactic presentation, initial session as 45
difficult clients. *See* challenging participants
diversity 13
divided attention 53–4
Division 12 (Society of Clinical Psychology) 1

early-warning system 173
eating disorders, MBCT and 4
eccentric clients, MBCT and 34–5
Ellis, Albert 128
Even the Rat Was White (Guthrie) 13
evidenced-based practices 58
exercises: body scan 73–8, 79–83, 175; eating raisins 68–72; mindfulness of breath 94; mindful stretching 107–8; modeling 25; rocks 184; sitting meditation 132, 145, 162; three-minute breathing space 104–5, 129; transitioning into 24; transitioning out of 25–6; unpleasant sensations 98
experienced mediators, MBCT and 34

fatigue 149
feedback 185–6
focus 53
free information sessions 45–6
fused thinking 57

giving, well-being and 52
group dynamics and interventions 14
groupies, MBCT and 36
group practice, confidentiality and 64
Guthrie, Robert 12–13

Happiness Trap, The (Harris) 163
Happy (film) 124
happy thoughts 67
Hayes, Stephen K. 93
Healing From Within (video) 116, 129, 141
health anxiety, MBCT and 4
health professionals, MBCT and 32
humor, stories and 29
hypnosis 57

initial information sessions: overview 45–6; session transcript 46–62
inquiry, three layers of 27–9

journaling 125
judgmental thinking 54, 141

Kabat-Zinn, Jon 2, 26, 53, 130, 183
Karate Kid, The (film) 178
knowing, two ways of 28

letting be: overview 131–2; session transcript 132–44
Linehan, Marsha 2

marketing, MBCT and 41
MBCT. *See* mindfulness-based cognitive therapy
mindful inquiry 26–9, 131
mindfulness: acceptance piece of 67; active, dynamic aspect of 54–5; attitudinal foundation of practice 26; benefits of 1; of breath 94; cultural representations of 52; exercises 24–6; Kabat-Zinn definition of 53; senses and 138
mindfulness-based cognitive therapy (MBCT): attitudinal foundation of 26; awareness and autopilot 63–4; basic qualifications 12–15; certification process 11–12; challenging participants 30–8; for children 14; defined 1; effectiveness of 2; exercises 24–6; increasing attention to 1–2; the language of 23–4; maintenance of competence 21–2; mindful inquiry 26–9; origins of 2; overview 4–7; personal practice of 19–21; practice practicalities 39–42; preparation for group 40; psychotherapy and 42; resources 15–19, 61; secular nature of 23; self-disclosure 30; self-sustaining nature of 182; stories and humor in 29; and traditional CBT 2–4; training and supervision 11–12, 15, 38–9; varieties of 4
mindfulness-based relapse prevention 37–8
mindfulness-based stress reduction (MBSR) 1, 2, 12
mindfulness exercises 24–6, 107–8
Mindfulness Meditation for Pain Relief (Kabat-Zinn) 101
mindfulness of breath 94

mindfulness practice, attitudinal foundation of 26
mindful stretching exercise 107–8
modeling 39
momentum 171, 175, 182
mood state-dependent memory 3

naysayers, MBCT and 35
negative thinking 2, 145
negative thought hit parade 125
noticing 27, 28, 59, 73, 102, 118

ongoing groups, MBCT and 42
orientation association area (brain) 52

pain 99–101
paradoxical strategic intervention effect 45
participant feedback 185–6
paying attention 53–4, 110–11
Peace in Every Step (Thich Nhat Hanh) 112
performance, stress and 48–50
personal practice 15, 19–21
physical sensation, staying present with 97–8
pleasant memories 93–4
posttraumatic stress disorder, MBCT and 4, 14–15, 23–4, 38
practice practicalities 39–42
preparation for group, MBCT and 40
present moment 54
procrastination 181
psychology, history of 13
psychotherapy, MBCT and 42, 64

raisin exercise 68–72
recordkeeping, MBCT and 42
reimbursement options, MBCT and 41–2
relapse prevention 14
relapse prevention plan 173
relaxation methods 57–8
resources 61
response flexibility 1
rock exercise 184

Sapolsky, Robert 89
scattered minds, gathering: overview 97–8; session transcript 98–115
scheduled worry 134
Segal, Zindel 1, 2

self-care 15, 19–21, 140; overview 161; session transcript 161–74
self-disclosure 30
Semple, Randye 21
sensations, changing nature of 97
senses, mindfulness and 138
serenity prayer 183
setting, MBCT and 39–40
Siddhartha Gautama 52
silent clients, MBCT and 36
sitting meditation 132, 145, 162
situational awareness 24
social justice 13
staying present: overview 116; session transcript 116–30
stories and humor 29
stress, MBCT and 45–6, 56–7
stress curve *48*
stress response, performance and 48–50
stretching exercises 109–10
stuck in the future, MBCT and 37
stuck in the past, MBCT and 36–7
student training and supervision 38–9
"Summer Day, The" (Oliver) 162
swimming pool analogy 112

taking notice, well-being and 50–1
Teasdale, John 2
thinking and feeling 28, 55–6
thought patterns, automatic and maladaptive 4
thoughts and facts: overview 145; session transcript 145–60
three-minute breathing space 104–5, 129
Tibetan bells *146*, 162
time management, MBCT and 40
tinnitus, MBCT and 4
traumas, MBCT and 38

uncoupling 28
Unpleasant Events Calendar 97
unpleasant sensations 98

walking meditation 112, 162
Watts, Alan 51, 67
well-being, five areas of 50–1
Williams, Mark 2
worry, scheduled 134

yoga 109

About the Author

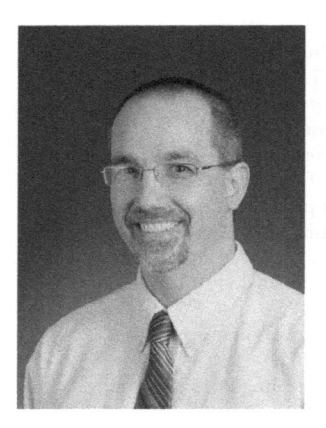

Richard W. Sears, Psy.D., Ph.D., M.B.A., A.B.P.P., is a board-certified clinical psychologist in Cincinnati, Ohio, where he conducts a private psychology and consultation practice. He regularly travels to present MBCT and mindfulness workshops to clinicians and the general public.

Dr. Sears is core faculty in the Psy.D. program at Union Institute & University and director of the Center for Clinical Mindfulness & Meditation. He is also clinical/research faculty at the University of Cincinnati Center for Integrative Health and Wellness and clinical assistant professor at Wright State University School of Professional Psychology. He is a psychologist contractor with Alliance Integrative Medicine and the Cincinnati VA Medical Center, where he is conducting research on MBCT. He is also volunteer associate professor of clinical psychiatry and behavioral neurosciences with UC College of Medicine, working with Dr. Sian Cotton and Dr. Melissa DelBello at Cincinnati Children's Hospital on projects involving mindfulness.

Dr. Sears is author of *Mindfulness: Living Through Challenges and Enriching Your Life in this Moment*, *Mindfulness in Clinical Practice* (with Dennis Tirch and Robert Denton), *Mindfulness-Based Cognitive Therapy for PTSD* (with Kathleen Chard), and *Consultation Skills for Mental Health Professionals* (with John Rudisill and Carrie Mason-Sears). He is editor of the book *Perspectives on Spirituality and Religion in Psychotherapy* (with Alison Niblick).

A fifth-degree black belt in To-Shin Do Ninja Martial Arts, Dr. Sears once served briefly as a personal protection agent for the Dalai Lama with his teacher, Stephen K. Hayes. He has practiced and taught mindfulness for more than 30 years, and received a Ph.D. in Buddhist Philosophy from Buddha Dharma University. He has been granted ordination in three Eastern wisdom traditions, and authority to teach Zen koans (*inka*) under Paul Wonji Lynch in the Zen lineage of Seung Sahn. Dr. Sears's website is www.psych-insights.com.

Lightning Source UK Ltd.
Milton Keynes UK
UKHW02f2029270418
321779UK00005B/163/P